Fashion Photography
Next

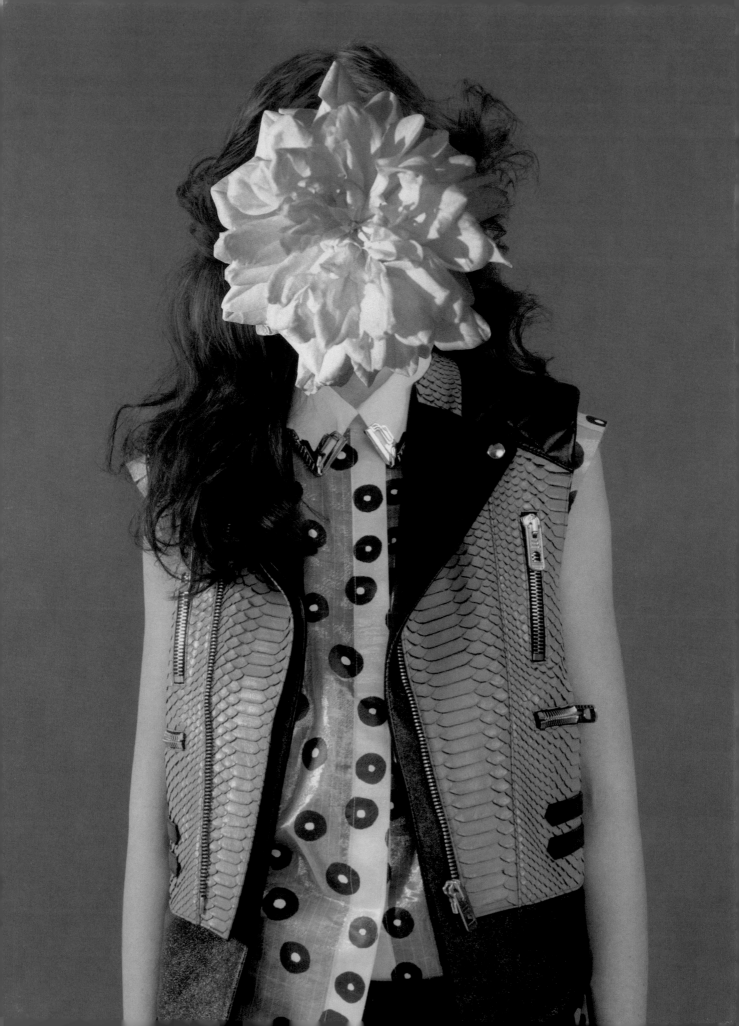

—

Fashion
Photography
Next

Magdalene Keaney

with contributions by Eleanor Weber

—

**with 272 illustrations,
208 in colour**

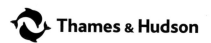
Thames & Hudson

———

The following sections were
researched and written
by Eleanor Weber:
Brendan Baker & Daniel Evans
Kasia Bobula
Timur Celikdag
Jonathan Hallam
Samuel Hodge
Chad Moore
Hanna Putz
Dennis Schoenberg
Saga Sig
Philippe Vogelenzang
Chardchakaj Waikawee
Ruvan Wijesooriya

———

Frontispiece: Mel Bles, Balenciaga Special with Linder Sterling, *Pop*, 2011.
Courtesy Stuart Shave / Modern Art, London.

First published in the United Kingdom in 2014
by Thames & Hudson Ltd, 181A High Holborn, London WC1V 7QX

Fashion Photography Next © 2014 Magdalene Keaney

All photographs © 2014 the individual photographers

Designed by Barnbrook

British Library Cataloguing-in-Publication Data
A catalogue record for this book is available from the British Library.

ISBN 978-0-500-54435-8

Printed and bound in China by C&C Offset Printing Co Ltd

To find out about all our publications, please visit
www.thamesandhudson.com
There you can subscribe to our e-newsletter, browse or download
our current catalogue, and buy any titles that are in print.

———

Table of Contents

———

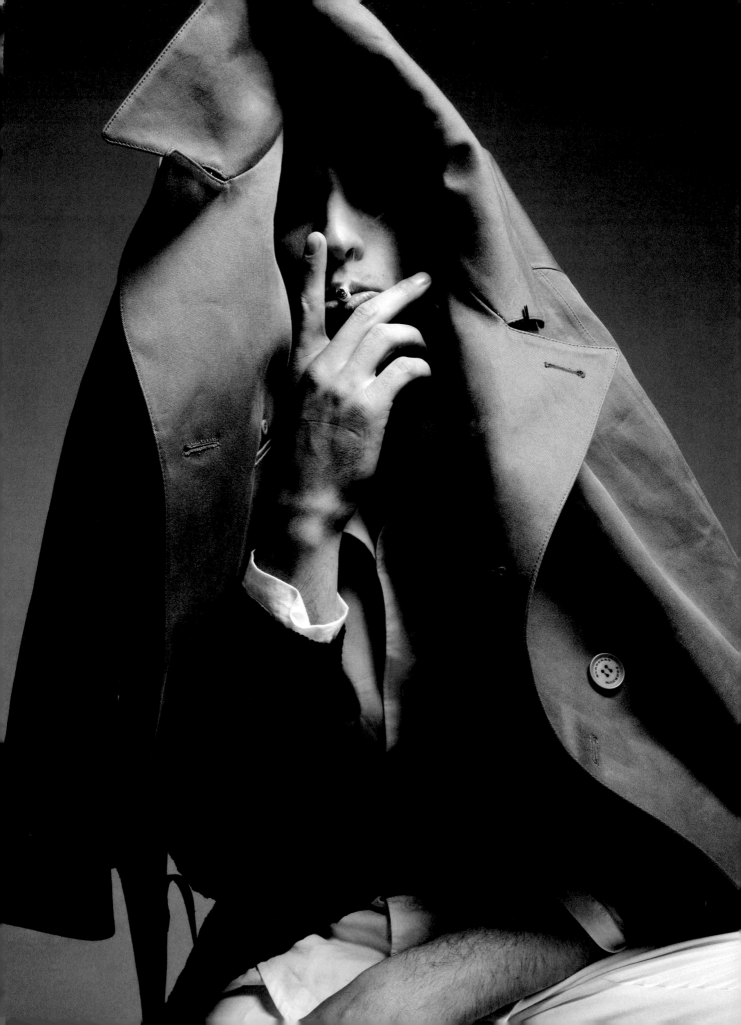

Photography Fashion

'It is much easier to decide outright that everything about the garb of an age is absolutely ugly than to devote oneself to the task of distilling from it the mysterious element of beauty that it may contain, however slight or minimal that element may be.'

Charles Baudelaire[1]

Would you be surprised if I told you that it is a little over a hundred years since fashion photographs began to appear in magazines? Did you imagine it was more or less? Though it's a century, a milestone provoking a natural tendency for retrospective consideration, the question may strike you as irrelevant. Fashion photography is probably something you think about in relation to the present, which actually makes a lot of sense. I'd like to talk about the present, but in reflecting on where we are now, let us begin by acknowledging that fashion photography also has a past and a future.

It is not my intention here to rehash the erudite accounts produced by significant commentators on the history of the fashion photograph. This book includes a list of further reading as a broad guide for those seeking more information. It is relevant to note, however, that these studies have been written from the perspective of both photographic history and theory as well as fashion history and theory, and organized in various ways: by individual artist; by time period; by stylistic or thematic approach; or by designer or fashion magazine. It is also worth pausing to consider the rather

momentous progression – the sheer volume and ground covered by fashion photography – since 1911, when Edward Steichen claimed to have made 'the first serious fashion photographs ever' for the French publication *Art et Décoration*.[2] Two years later, in January 1913, a fashion photograph appeared in US *Vogue*, arguably for the first time. A 'fashion portrait' of Gertrude Vanderbilt Whitney, it was taken by Adolph de Meyer, the magazine's first staff photographer.[3]

Our world is constantly changing. Fashion photography has always been concerned with describing and situating change, a project that is certainly precipitated by the expectation of the new – new seasons, new collections, new editorial and new advertising in the next new issue of a magazine. But fashion photography has also meaningfully responded to newness in contemporary life – changes in social structures, economic circumstances or gender expectations – as well as to new developments, both practical and theoretical, in photography and the visual arts. Many stylistic developments in the history of photography are linked to technological progression, with smaller cameras, faster films, artificial lights, chemical processing and colour film all

facilitating a wider range of creative choices. Fashion photography has always quickly embraced the possibilities offered by the latest technology. Aided by commercial advertising budgets and imperatives, it has led the platform development of digital image capture and post-production in a far more sustained and sophisticated way than other non-commercial genres. The potential to retouch an image should not be thought of as a prerogative of the 'digital age' (post-1990), or of the fashion photograph in particular. That said, the fashion-driven inclination to push the boundaries of digital image-making further, more quickly, and the processes demanded by the film-less capture and seamless retouching implemented in the fashion industry during the late 1990s and early 2000s, certainly revolutionized the act of taking a photograph. These developments in photographic hardware and software were subsequently made available to and used by non-commercial photographers.

The past, present and future of fashion photography are, of course, linked, though this is not to suggest a neat linear march of the 'next' conveniently building on the 'last' to get to the 'now'. The evolution of the fashion image is an important part of the photographic canon and the history of visual culture in general, even when this has been uncomfortable, undesirable or difficult to articulate – be it because of the shifting status of photography itself, because of the contested validity of presenting fashion photographs outside a fashion framework, or because of convention and status quo.

The first premise of this book is that fashion photographers are first and foremost *photographers*. It will explore a new generation of image-makers working with fashion who are necessarily *photographers first*. Though characterized as 'new generation' or 'emerging', they are not specifically linked by their age; rather, they share a creative vision with a distinct momentum towards the future. I have been interested in identifying the conceptual and stylistic markers that define where contemporary fashion photography is at, as well as in discovering the practitioners producing groundbreaking work aside from the establishment figures – i.e. the leading photographers who continue to set agendas and produce innovative and influential work, but have already been extensively documented and discussed. (This latter group might include photographers who were themselves emerging during the 1980s and '90s, such as Inez and Vinoodh, Nick Knight, Craig McDean, Steven Meisel, Mert and Marcus, Terry Richardson, Mario Sorrenti, David Sims, Juergen Teller, Mario Testino and Wolfgang Tillmans.) *Fashion Photography Next* is therefore an optimistic platform for the photographers whose work is not widely known outside of industry experts, but should be.

In thinking about this proposition, there is a basic linguistic issue at work that needs to be teased out: the placement of the word 'fashion' in front of the word 'photography'. In some ways, this ordering is perfectly sensible. We use words to classify and describe things and all the photographers featured in this book include fashion in their work in a way that adds meaning to the images, and/or their images are displayed in fashion contexts, mostly on the printed page of a magazine. And yet when it comes to fashion photography, rarely in the cultural and historical analysis of the medium has such a sustained dismissive emphasis been placed on that first word. For example, one might define Julia Margaret Cameron, Cindy Sherman or Rineke Dijkstra as portrait photographers, despite the fact that this is a very generalized description. While at one time they might have been discounted as women photographers, they are not marginalized as portrait photographers. The same point applies with the genre descriptions of landscape, still life or nude, although these traditional boundaries or definitions are becoming increasingly malleable and incompatible with much contemporary practice. In his book *Hiding*, Mark C. Taylor reminds us that the very things that make fashion attractive to us also make it appear insubstantial: 'On the one hand to label something fashionable is to embrace it as smart, sophisticated, elegant, current and timely. On the other hand, to characterize something as fashionable is to dismiss it as trendy, trivial, inconsequential, insignificant and fleeting.'[4] It is as though the very word that describes it also undermines it.

Sticking with the past, it seems to me that there have been two predominant ways in which we are comfortable dealing with and accepting fashion photography as a credible photographic contribution. One is when it is collected and exhibited by a national or state-run art gallery or museum, so that the image or image-maker is given institutional legitimacy. The other is as we move further away from the time a fashion photograph was taken, so by a retrospective process of historical legitimacy.

Both of these outmoded paradigms rely on complex external processes that are sometimes evoked in order to discuss the fashion photograph as 'art'. But the justification or forced contextualization of fashion photography as art is as irrelevant and meaningless as at the other extreme: relegating it to the status of ephemera or commerce alone. This fashion / art / photography debate diverts us from the possibility of considering a fashion image without apology, and without trying to make it something it is not and does not need to be.

In other words, when examining this selection of new generation work, made by practitioners who are first and foremost photographers, let us accept two more basic premises: that fashion photography has its own unique values and characteristics; and that these values and characteristics are not dependent on anything other than the values and characteristics of fashion photography itself. Then, remembering the power held by one word preceding another, let us put the word 'photography' before the word 'fashion' and consider what it might mean to say *Photography Fashion*.

'Remembering the power held by one word preceding another, let us put the word "photography" before the word "fashion" and consider what it might mean to say *Photography Fashion*.'

Perhaps it has taken the past century to get to the point where we are able to do this. Perhaps it is only possible to talk confidently about fashion photography on its own terms since the relatively recent establishment of structures around its production and dissemination: the discourses and debates that have arisen over the last few decades in fashion-related publications and exhibitions, for example, or the growing number of university courses in fashion photography. Technically speaking, an anonymous catalogue photograph of a garment on an online fashion boutique is a fashion photograph, just as a passport photograph is also a portrait. This book is not concerned with the ubiquitous intersection of photography and fashion, however. It does not declare that all fashion photography is of equal value, nor does it argue that the value of images does not shift or alter. Instead, it asks what distinguishes a particular photographer working with or around fashion today as notable?

In recent years, some commentators have lamented the state of fashion image-making as derivative and limited by commercial imperatives. To a degree, this may be true. In response to such claims, my research for *Fashion Photography Next* has been conceptualized as an open-ended question or experiment. Was it possible to identify a group of photographers that warranted discussion? What were the recurring issues, approaches or concerns, if any, shared in their work? When presented collectively, would there be an obvious generational shift from the established practitioners? Were traditional definitions such as still life or portrait, studio or location, and paradigms such as nationality and gender, still relevant? Would new ways of organizing such a group, and of thinking about structural relationships, become apparent?

Variance and hybridity have emerged as two of the defining themes of this book. More than ever before, there is less of a sense of homogeneity around the production of fashion imagery – technically, stylistically, conceptually, and even in the way one might go about being a fashion photographer. Contrary to what you might expect, the institution of the paper-based magazine as

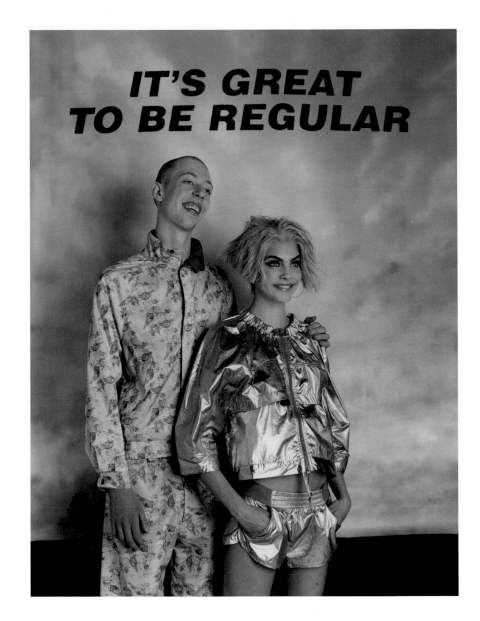

IT'S GREAT TO BE REGULAR

the primary commissioner of fashion editorial remains dominant, and I for one doubt that it will ever disappear. History has shown us that the precarity of fashion publishing is not limited to our time, nor is it connected to advancements in technology. *Vanity Fair* folded between 1936 and 1981, for example, and the well-known British magazine *Nova* lasted only ten years, from 1965 to 1975. While *The Face* – one of the most important magazines for the photographers in this book (with *i-D* being the other key influence) – was finally closed in 2004 after twenty-four years, printed fashion periodicals continue to appear on newsstands. These include relatively new forces such as *The Gentlewoman*, *PonyStep*, *Under/Current*, *Acne Paper*, *The Room* and the Condé Nast-owned *Love*, as well as the longer standing fashion publications *032c*, *Purple*, *Pop*, *Arena Homme +*, *V* and *W*.

Of course, many of these magazines simultaneously maintain digital platforms. The most effective of these sites are not an attempt to reproduce the printed version online; instead, they offer a specific Web-based experience that can include film and moving image, 'behind the scenes' specials and links to social media, chat sites and blogs. For example, *Dazed Digital*, the online edition of *Dazed&Confused*, is filled with a sense of hyperactive energy and almost excessive stimulation. Covering music, fashion, art, film and photography, with images and headings running both horizontally and vertically, the website is responsive, fast-paced, all there, all at once. 'Click for Fashion Week's Hottest' and 'Stand to Attention' it bids its readers, offering them 'the latest', 'the brightest', 'the best' and 'the most viewed'. Connect to Twitter, Tumblr, YouTube, Instagram and Facebook;

See, Hear, Enter, Subscribe, Like, Comment, Share, Post, Mix, Remix and, of course, Buy the New Issue.

Having said this, the global prevalence of underground, independent or self-publishing – resulting from both digital platforms and economic recession – has to some degree diluted the monopoly of the large paper-based publishing houses and magazine mastheads, providing image-makers and their audience with an alternative. This tends to operate on a more localized level because of smaller or limited-edition print runs and distribution issues, as well as the absolutely overwhelming density of images and text on the Web.[5] Outside of the more mainstream websites and publications, these blogs or zines are most likely found if you know about them first, reinforcing the notion of the specialized audience and emphasizing the importance of knowledge exchange at a local or community level. For example, you might walk past an issue of the free magazine *Beat*, which commissions many leading fashion photographers, at various London outlets but not think to pick it up unless you have a particular interest in indie music or street style.[6] And *Beat* magazine might only be stocked in shops targeting a specific age or demographic within a particular area of the city. This example highlights the development of a double or parallel trajectory of fashion image-making, with photographers working between a regional or communal circuit and the brand-led international fashion industry. The two strands have different values and ideas about what makes a good fashion photograph: experimentation and mistakes might be accepted or even encouraged in the first, for instance, but not in the second.

Independent or self-publishing have also resulted in a healthy re-evaluation of the previous neediness of many emerging fashion photographers for vindication by the gallery or exhibition system. Many of the photographers featured here have made their own books or worked with independent publishers, including Samuel Hodge (*Sometimes I Just Need Quiet*, 2008), Jamie Hawkesworth (*Preston Bus Station*, 2010), Tyrone Lebon (*Nothing Lasts Forever*, 2011), Daniel Evans (*3 Months in Another Place*, 2011), Chad Moore (*Between Us*, 2011), Charlie Engman (*Field*, 2011), Erik Madigan Heck (*January to August*, 2011) and Clare Shilland (*Love From Alice*, 2011). If these publications generate an audience and are reviewed, promoted and discussed online – sometimes even selling out – then the expense and difficulty of procuring a gallery space and hanging prints on a wall does seem redundant. That is unless the collaborative or installation potential of the exhibition venue or organization can offer other significant creative opportunities, pleasures or exposure.

Two important points are worth noting here. Firstly, the ever-increasing range of opportunities in the public sphere for fashion photographers to get work has broken down the traditional 'apprenticeship' training structure. There are now alternative routes into fashion photography besides assisting an established name for a number of years, which has enabled a greater diversity of practitioners in the industry. So, for example, while Daniel Jackson assisted the enormously influential David Sims (just as Sims himself assisted Robert Erdmann and Norman Watson), or Jermaine Francis spent a period with Corinne Day, or Boo George worked with Julian Broad, Harley Weir is a self-taught photographer who

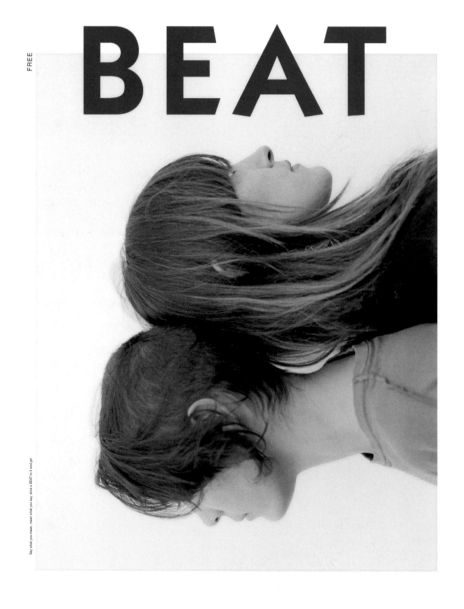

FREE

BEAT

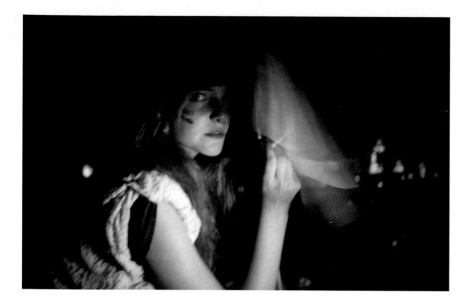

began her successful career in editorial after *Vice* magazine spotted her work on Flickr.[7] Similarly, Charlie Engman's break on *Dazed Digital* came on the strength of some personal images he posted on Flickr that were a by-product of one of his sculptural projects at university.[8] The proliferation of photography courses at college or university level has also undoubtedly shaped the scope of who might begin to make fashion images, and how or why they might do this. The majority of the photographers discussed here studied photography, or art and design-related subjects, at university. For better or worse, many universities are now offering bachelor's and master's degrees in fashion photography, though the effects of these more specific courses are not yet measurable or reliably visible.

Secondly, the rule of the centre still holds: London and New York, and to a lesser extent Paris, remain the living and working bases for most of the photographers in this book. Apart from Chardchakaj Waikawee in Thailand and Samuel Hodge in Australia, the remainder of the photographers are based in Europe and the US. While mastheads such as *Vogue* and *Harper's Bazaar* have taken off in fast-growing Asian economies such as China and India, in general main fashion stories are still produced with photographers in London and New York, rather than by local talent.

All of the work featured in this book is made with a nuanced understanding of the critical debates surrounding fashion photography and a knowledge of the

history of photography, fashion or otherwise. The 'realist' approach, for example, which draws on documentary or diaristic traditions, is still an important starting-point for many photographers, as is the psychological or fictional fashion narrative, which is heavily influenced by film. Both are long-standing precedents in the making of the fashion image.

Fashion photographs still fit into categories. They may be studio or location-based, for instance, though the definition of the studio and the way in which 'studio' images are made has changed considerably, even in the last ten years. On a practical level, this is because digital image capture has dramatically altered equipment and apparatus, including cameras, to the extent that a digital operator is often a key member of the photographic team. Photographers are now able to see and edit their images on screen immediately after taking the shots. More abstractly, the photographic studio can simultaneously be both a real and a virtual performance and working space, as well as an imaginary arena created after the shoot during post-production. While practitioners may appear to work within a specific genre – such as portraiture, for example, which has a particularly strong lineage in the history of fashion photography – this is rarely a pure or exclusive engagement. An image sequence or story, and sometimes even a single photograph, can incorporate portrait, still-life, landscape, abstract and conceptual, as well as studio or location-based, approaches. Perhaps this can be understood as the visual equivalent of the

music sample, mash-up, sound bite or remix that is so prevalent in contemporary culture.

The use of realist aesthetics in fashion photography as a means of social comment and even political agitation has been the focus of excellent written analysis and curatorial consideration, and can be traced back to the 1940s (although was probably most significant during the periods of economic recession in the UK in the 1980s and '90s). Cultural and social issues such as race, sexuality, class, age, disempowerment, boredom, individuality, austerity and recession, and community are not new subjects for photographers and continue to be important preoccupations. These critical concerns have extended and shifted with the issues that are pressing to our time to incorporate questions of sustainability and consumption, corporate psychology versus local thinking, increasing financial inequality, and the pervasiveness of surveillance in our lives.

My co-contributor, Eleanor Weber, has succinctly articulated a further shift, explaining that central to the thread of realist fashion image-making for the newer 'socially networked' generation is the figure of the photographer '*living* in this time, not merely recording it'. '"No-technique" images have become symbolic of the time we live in,' she says. 'Their sense of fast, rebellious, carefree youthfulness captures the essence

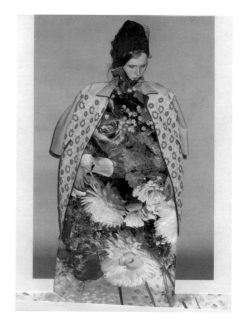

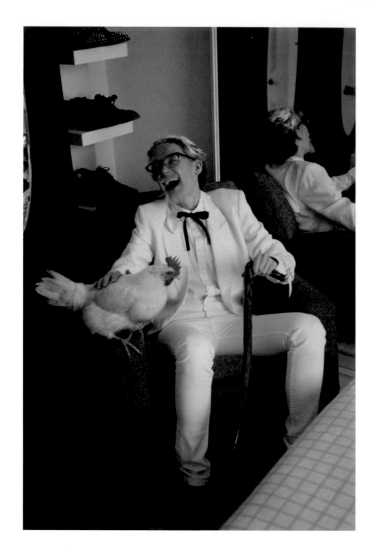

'Each photographer contributes to our awareness of the importance of fashion imagery as a vital and dynamic site of progressive ideas and debates.'

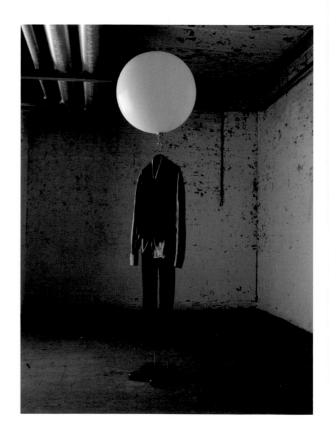

6 Daniel Jackson, 'Suits On', *AnOther Man*, 2011 — 9 Tyrone Lebon, 'Frank and Cara', *i-D*, 2012 — 10 Clare Shilland, 'Warpaint', *Beat*, 2010

11 above Chad Moore, 'Imogen (Flag)', 2010 — 11 below Charlie Engman, 'Sketch with pink and florals', 2012 — 12 left Samuel Hodge, 'The Curse of the Colonel', 2012

12 right Jacob Sutton, 'Powder', *Mixte*, 2007 — 13 Jonathan Hallam, 'Rêve du situationnisme', *French*, 2009

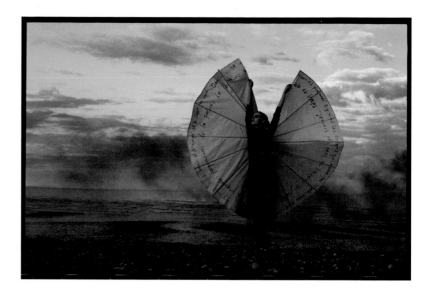

of a society that wants to know everything about everyone, where anyone can be a celebrity, and where the lines between model, socialite, musician, actress, artist and "icon" are ever more blurred… Whether the aim is portrait or fashion image is irrelevant; from a new vantage of integrated genres the photographer is simultaneously capturing and creating the zeitgeist.'[9]

An emphasis on play is another important trend, with many photographers creating clever and witty images that transform fashion photographs – quite wonderfully at times – into tableaux, performances or visual puns. Fashion film is not the focus of this book but must be mentioned as many contemporary photographers often make still and moving images simultaneously; I would argue that this has influenced approaches to movement and pose in the studio.[10] The continued prevalence of the directorial or cinematographic approach to still production through the conceptualization, casting, styling and sequencing of images is more relevant here. Contemporary fashion stories sometimes span twenty to thirty pages in a magazine, allowing complex and often obscure narratives and characters to develop.

A significant number of emerging fashion photographers prioritize materiality and medium-based issues in their images, something that is perhaps surprising in today's era, when we might assume that the adherence would be to digital methods. While the mid-2000s felt like the inevitable endpoint for analogue fashion photography, which was then the preserve of only the most important and powerful photographers, many present-day practitioners work with film and Polaroid, both as a creative choice

and as an act of resistance to the commercial and client pressure to shoot digital. Consequently, after the increasingly startling, extreme and ubiquitous retouching of the first decade of the twenty-first century, we can now see a return to darkroom processing and minimal post-production. Some photographers consciously draw attention to the artifice of the fashion image, questioning the limits of the medium by intervening with deliberately lo-fi, hand-drawn illustrations, by collaging together digital and analogue photographs, or by mixing in-camera effects with post-production – whatever achieves the desired creative or conceptual result. Others reject the seamlessness of digital but not the platform itself by pushing artificiality further, pursuing a digital hyperreality and proposing experimental notions of beauty and picture-making. When it comes to the way in which fashion photographs are created, the rule, it would seem, is that there are no rules.

Fashion photography's engagement with the body will always provoke debates about sexuality and gender roles. There is a further need, however, to look beyond the image frame and address the issue of who is taking the photograph. One of the biggest shifts in the last decade is that there are now more women making fashion images. While I am not suggesting that their work has any kind of inherent feminine style or quality, these women photographing women – and, significantly, women photographing men – offer a different perspective by simple virtue of the fact that in the past the genre has been dominated by male practitioners.

Fashion Photography Next began with an observation about the confidence and vigour of a group of photographers whose work deserves more recognition outside the industry. Photographers whose technical, stylistic, compositional, subject-based or conceptual approaches are unapologetic, original, relevant, influential, sophisticated, unexpected, playful, thought-provoking and transformative. Each one contributes to our awareness of the importance of fashion imagery – within contemporary photographic practice and global culture more broadly – as a vital and dynamic site of progressive ideas and debates.

[1] Charles Baudelaire (1863), 'The Painter of Modern Life' in *The Painter of Modern Life and Other Essays,* London: Phaidon, 1995.

[2] Steichen's images of Poiret fashions were published in *Art et Décoration* in April 1911. See Chapter 7 in Edward Steichen, *A Life in Photography*, New York: Bonanza Books, 1984.

[3] Norberto Angeletti and Alberto Oliva, *In Vogue: An Illustrated History of the World's Most Famous Fashion Magazine*, New York: Rizzoli, 2012.

[4] Mark C. Taylor, *Hiding,* University of Chicago Press, 1997, pp. 167– 68. With thanks to eX de Medici for bringing this important book to my attention.

[5] For instance, if you type 'fashion photography' into an internet search engine, the results would probably not include the majority of the photographers discussed in this book, even though they are some of the most significant practitioners in the industry today.

[6] *Beat* magazine is a biannual print publication that was founded by Hanna Hanra in 2010, and features art direction by Dean Langley.

[7] Harley Weir, 'Take Me To The Other Side', *Vice,* 2008, available at: www.vice.com/ en_uk / read / fashion-take-me-other-side-v15n2 [accessed February 2013]

[8] Charlie Engman and Hayley Caradoc-Hodgkins, 'Flickr Showcase: Charlie Engman', *Dazed Digital,* 2009, available at: www.dazeddigital.com / photography /article/ 3406 / 1 / flickr-showcase-charlie-engman [accessed May 2013]

[9] Eleanor Weber and Magdalene Keaney, 'The Model Portrait', unpublished essay, 2010.

[10] Contemporary fashion film is a complex genre. More and more photographers have started making moving images, facilitated by the technological advancements in cameras that allow still or moving images to be produced simultaneously or in conjunction with each other. Moving-image production, however, requires a very different set of creative and technical skills than still photography. In my opinion, the number of contemporary fashion films that might be viewed at best as necessary consequences of digital platform development, and at worst as responses to client demands, is far higher than the number of coherent, interesting, influential, innovative, challenging or relevant fashion films.

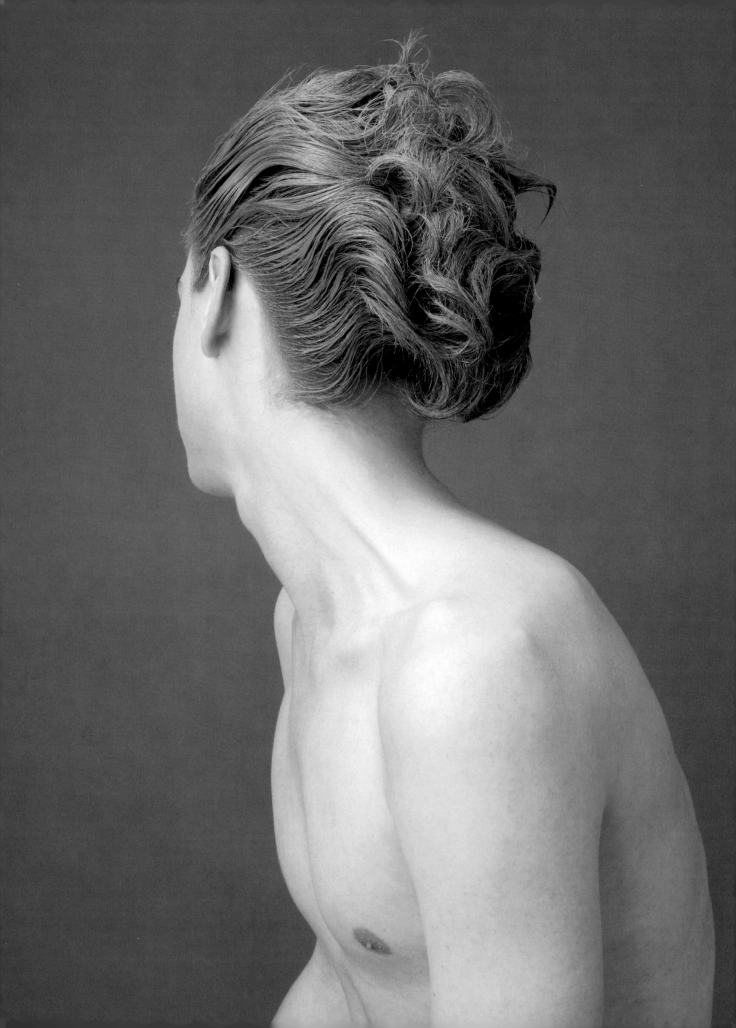

Brendan Baker and Daniel Evans's singular, twenty-first-century style has strong roots in post-internet culture.

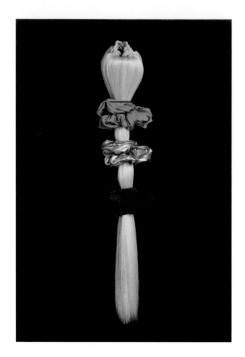

British photographers Brendan Baker (b. 1988) and Daniel Evans (b. 1990) both came to photography as teenagers, via skateboarding and graffiti respectively. They first met while studying photography at the University for the Creative Arts in Farnham, just outside London, where they were part of the same friendship group in their first year and shared a house with two other friends in their second year. Despite recognizing that they shared almost the same photographic interests and direction, with a similar level of motivation and desire to produce, Baker and Evans did not set out to work collaboratively and did not begin taking photographs together officially until their third year. At this time, they decided to work as a duo on a more focused project to solidify what had already begun to occur between them the year before as a much looser series of mutual experiments.

The results of this first project together were very well received. In their final year at university, Baker and Evans were selected for *Source* magazine's annual Graduate Photography Online showcase by Susan Bright, Tanya Kiang and Trish Lambe, and for *Wallpaper*'s 2012 Graduate Directory. Since graduating in 2011, they have continued to work together, mainly in a fashion context. Neither of them had originally intended to work in fashion – their fine art-centric undergraduate course is most famous for its roots in the classic British documentary photography tradition. Nevertheless, they found themselves drawn to fashion after a stylist approached them with the opportunity to work with *Pop* online magazine. More fashion work ensued, and their client list has expanded to include magazines such as *AnOther*,

Dazed & Confused, Nowness, Wonderland, Hotshoe, The Room and *Self Publish, Be Happy*, as well as MTV, Whistles, Y'OH, Topshop, among many others. In addition, they have exhibited their photographs across the UK, USA and India, including in the 2012 show 'Fresh Faced + Wild Eyed' at the Photographers' Gallery in London.

Usually working with digital cameras, Baker and Evans take turns shooting and directing, always bearing in mind where they want to go with a story, but without predetermining anything too rigidly. They say this is 'one of the advantages of working as a duo; there's always a dialogue going on between us about what we could change, what's good, what's bad and where we can take the idea'. Inspired by photographers such as Jason Evans and Viviane Sassen, the pair do not seek to distinguish between their fashion and personal work and there is little difference between these two sides of their practice. They see this consistency as a mark of their stylistic integrity.

Following in a line of famous photographic double acts that includes Inez and Vinoodh, and Mert and Marcus, Baker and Evans are carving out a very singular, twenty-first-century style that has strong roots in post-internet culture. Shot mainly in the studio using artificial lighting – mostly flash – their photographs have a sense of cool detachment without taking themselves too seriously. The composition and framing often serve to subtract the subjects from their original contexts so as to confound a conventional reading.

Baker describes his interest in the 'body as object', where the distinction between human and non-human is subordinate to the aim of creating 'something more akin to an abstract painting, something bold and visually exciting that is simply a joy to look at while also retaining some kind of substance and esotericism'. The images, which often feature limited colour palettes in order to emphasize form, generate multiple layers of interpretation. For example, in a 2013 photograph for *District MTV*, a seemingly banal hair extension is given a strange life through its exaggerated staging against a dramatic black background. It floats rootlessly, revealing the photographers' interest in Surrealism. This approach prevents the hair extension from serving its prescribed purpose as a fashion accessory and instead highlights the very oddness of its objecthood. We can identify a similar tactic in Baker and Evans's portrait photographs, in which sitters often seem to stare naively at the viewer in benign friendliness, reminding us of our ultimate disconnect from that which is captured photographically.

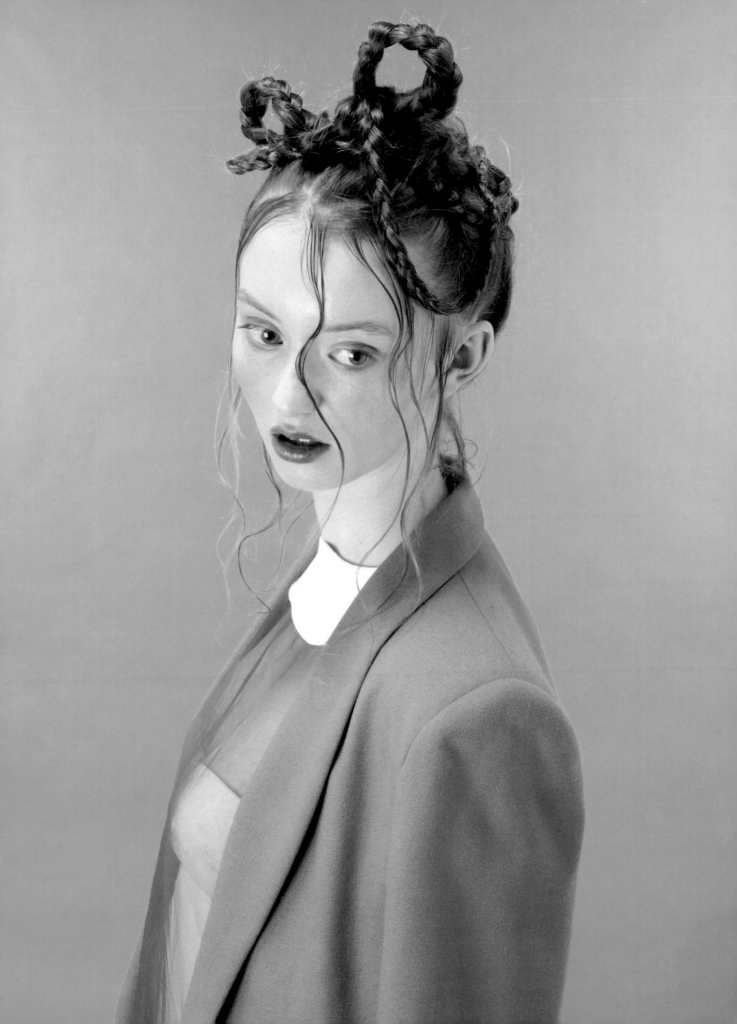

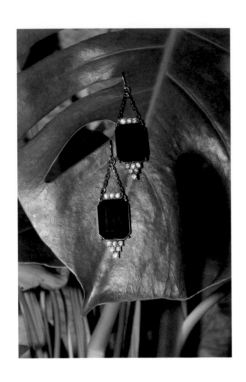

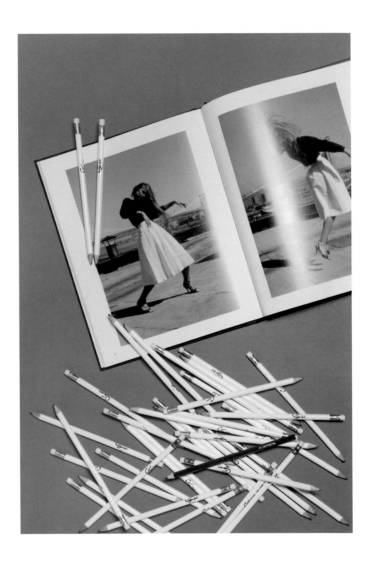

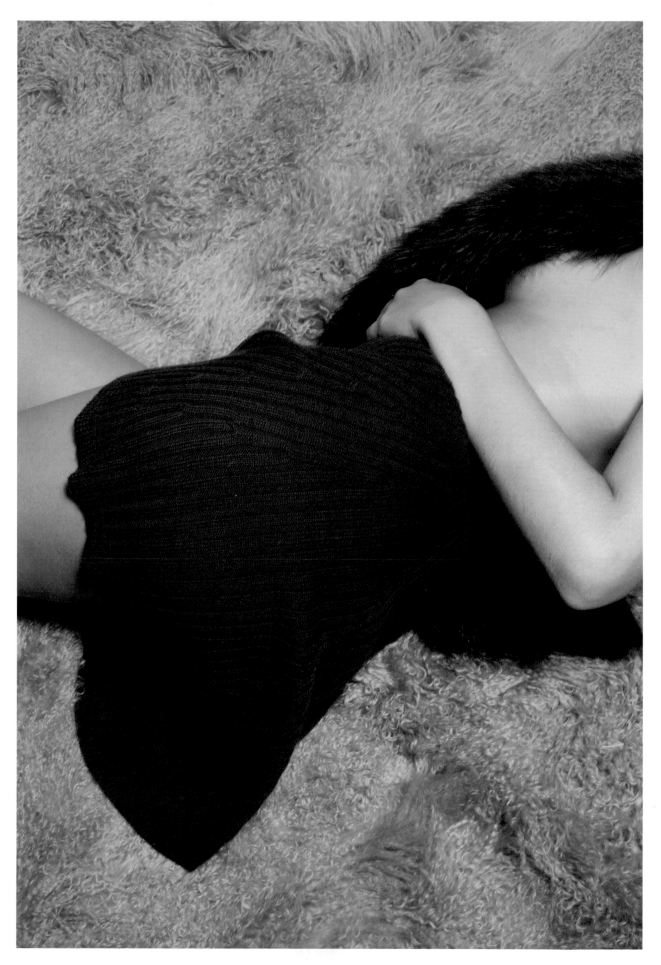

Brendan Baker & Daniel Evans

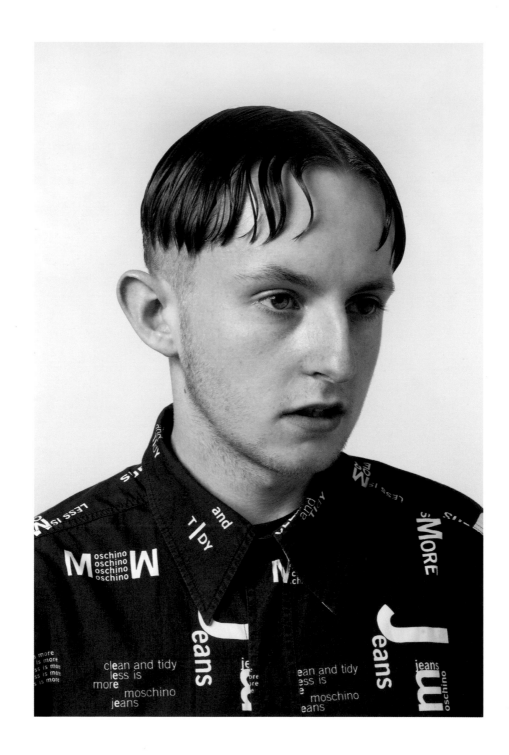

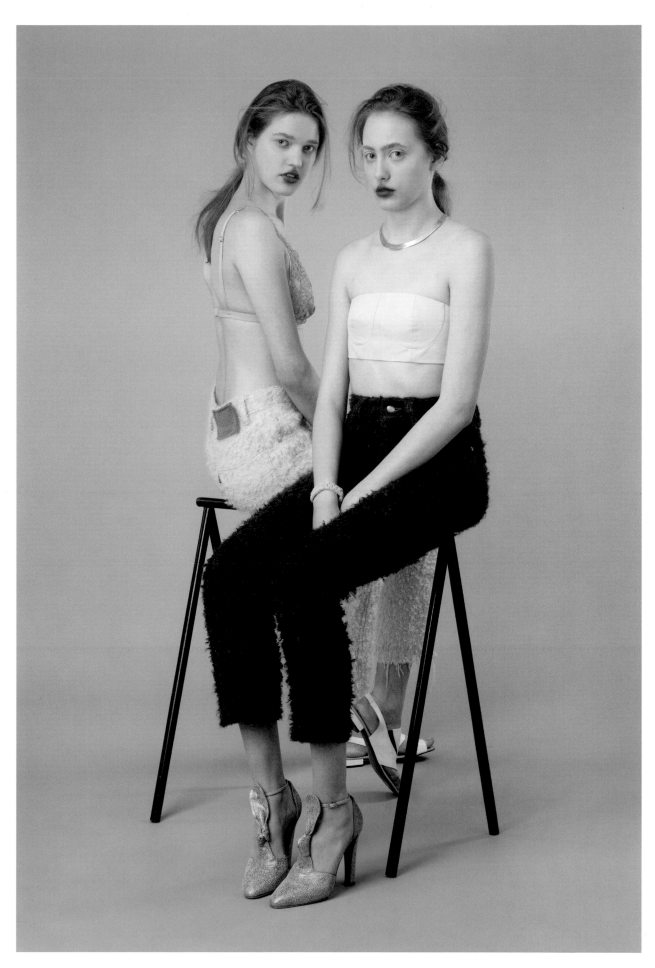

Brendan Baker & Daniel Evans

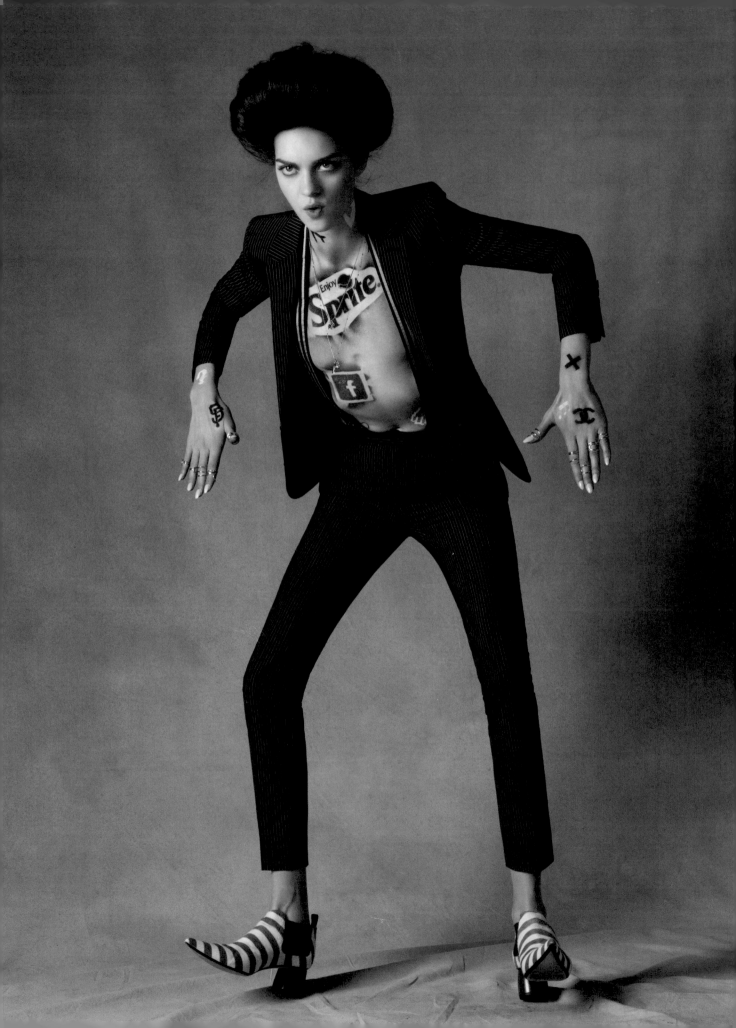

Mel Bles is a studio photographer but her images are rarely composed from a single frame.

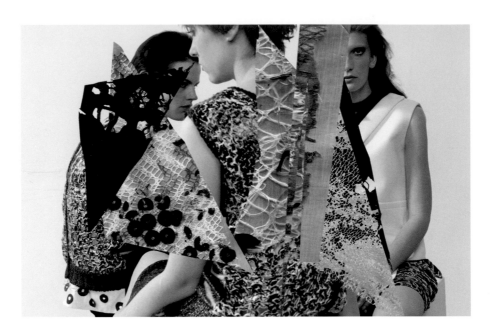

Mel Bles (b. 1978) lives and works in London. She studied graphic design at Central Saint Martins College of Art and Design, where she gravitated towards working with film and photography. Her approach to fashion image-making was in part shaped by British photographers William Selden and Benjamin Alexander Huseby, both of whom she assisted, as they emphasize the importance of developing a unique visual language. For Bles, this does not mean building up a repetitive uniformity, but rather avoiding the commercial pressure to create a new superficial style or theme with each commission.

The sense of continued innovation and movement in Bles's work – which does, in fact, often look very different from one story to the next – comes from her exploration of a range of photographic processes and ideas, including digital techniques, texture, colour blocks, three-dimensional form and, significantly, page layouts and image juxtapositions. In Bles's hands, the various images in a single story can appear quite diverse. She utilizes different modes of lighting or image resolution in such a way that often the photographs do not form a coherent narrative; rather, they follow one after another to create an overall impression of a visual whole.

Bles is primarily a studio photographer, although her finished images are rarely composed from a single frame. She makes sophisticated and precise use of digital hardware and software on set, where she not only shoots a still but also works on its treatment and place in a story. Since her first published portrait of American rap icon Timberland appeared in *Dazed & Confused* in 2008, Bles's editorial has quickly gained momentum. In recent seasons, she has become a tour de force among the prestigious London-based fashion biannuals *Pop*, *Arena Homme +*, *Exit* and *Under/Current*.

Bles's open and playful creative methods and her predilection for collage proved ideal in a 2011 Balenciaga special for *Pop*, for which she collaborated with artists Meredyth Sparks, Clunie Reid and Linder Sterling. In another project for *Pop*, also in 2011, she worked with renowned artist duo Lucy + Jorge Orta, whose cross-disciplinary practice investigates, among other things, the body in relation to the environment. Styled by Vanessa Reid around Céline garments, this story mixed studio photographs by Bles with computer-generated drawings by the Ortas, deconstructing the two-dimensional representation of women in fashion by attempting to structurally render or rebuild female bodies as three-dimensional sculptural forms. For the same project, Bles created highly saturated and pixelated landscapes as a counterpoint to some of the images. As in most of her editorials, the individual photographs are displayed across double pages, so the magazine layout is again of fundamental importance.

———

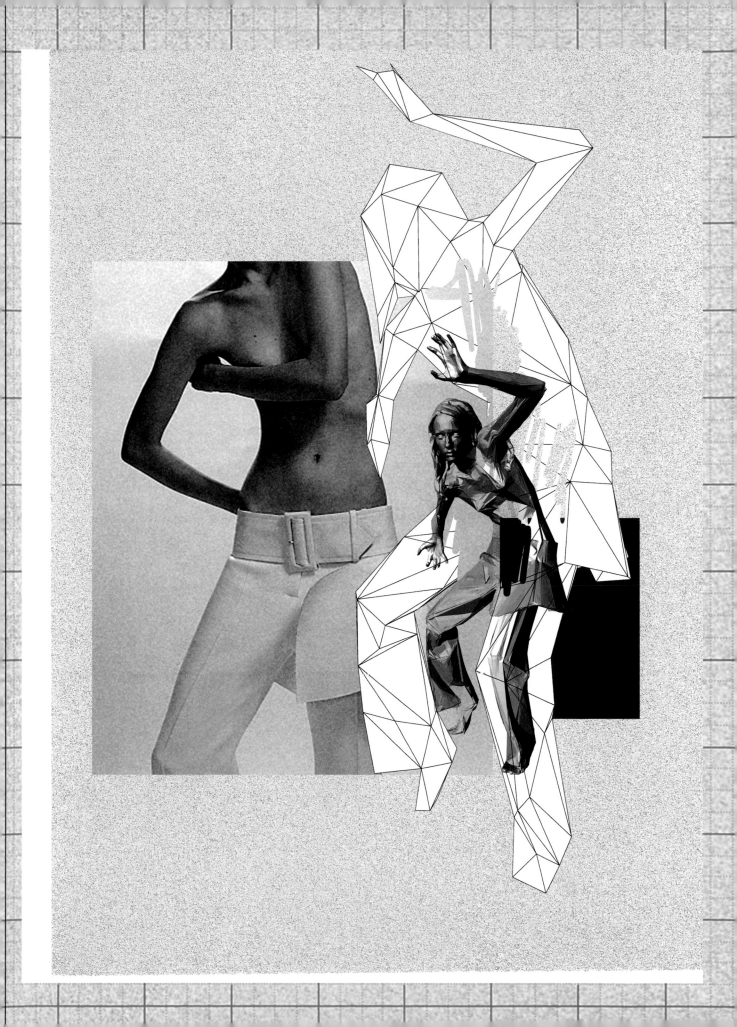

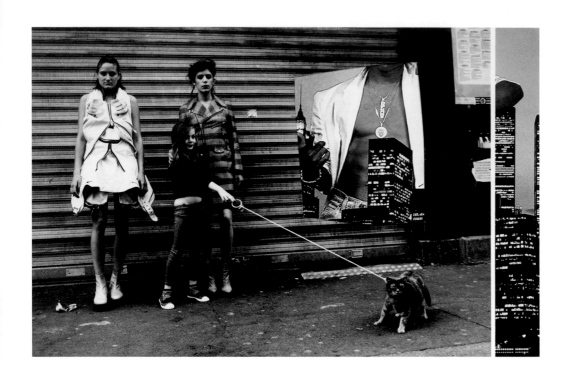

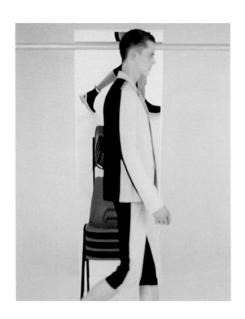

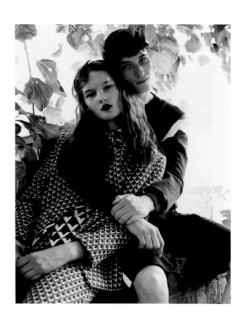

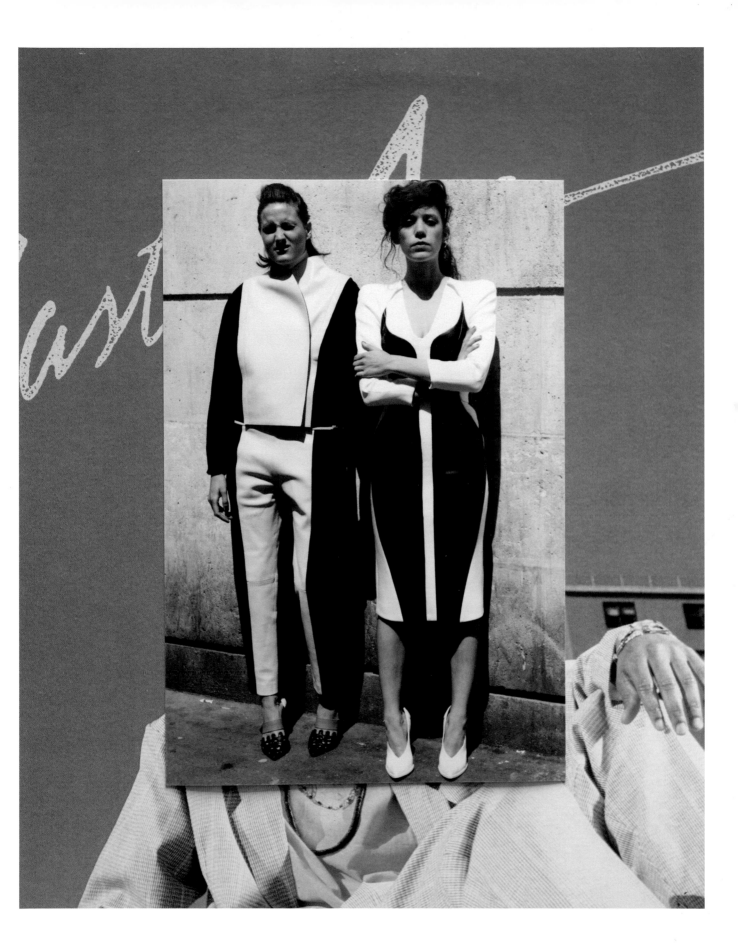

Mel Bles

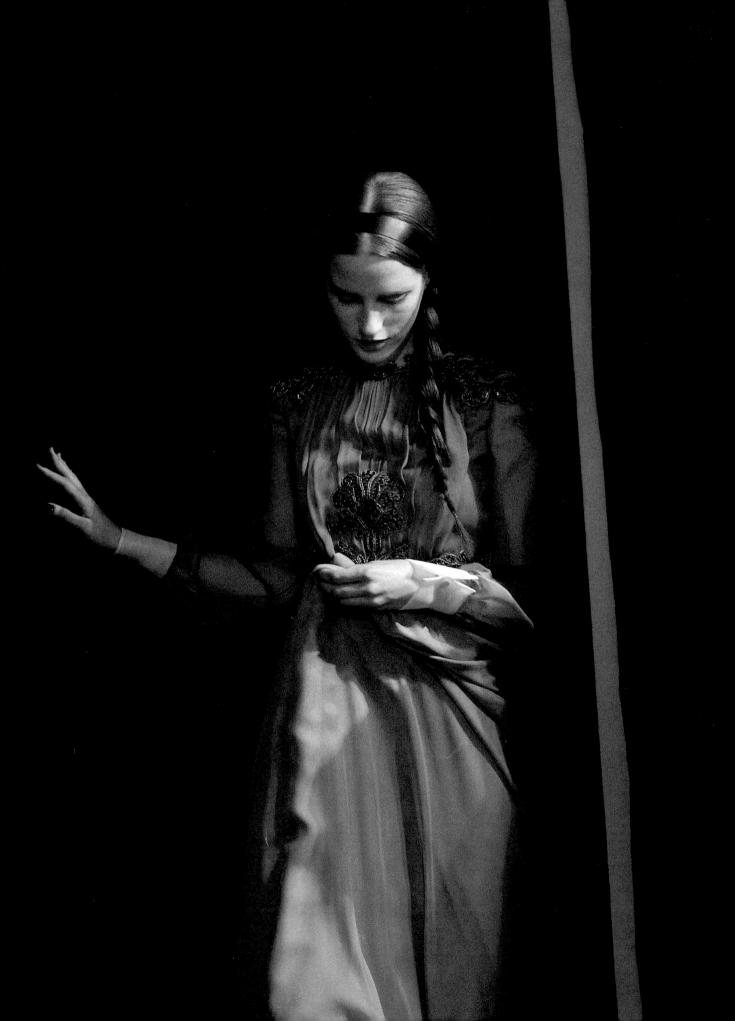

Kasia Bobula's backstage work is centred around the idea of the chance encounter.

Kasia Bobula

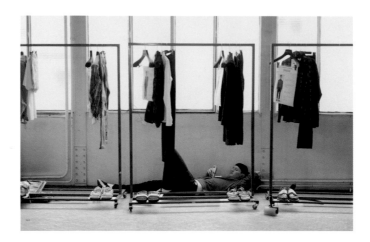

Kasia Bobula (b. 1983) grew up in Warsaw and is now based in London. In 2007, she graduated from Central Saint Martins College of Art and Design with a BA in fashion design and marketing. In February 2008, not long after finishing university, she was invited to take backstage photographs at a fashion show by a friend, the Polish designer Krystof Strozyna, who was setting up his own label. Strozyna liked Bobula's personal work and originally requested the images for his own documentation purposes. At the time, Bobula did not have a point-and-shoot camera and so used an old 35 mm SLR. As she recalls: 'I had no idea about the lighting backstage, no flash and only two rolls of film.' Despite her relative inexperience, the resulting images were compelling. She realized they held potential, the beginnings of a style that could be further explored.

Bobula decided to send the images to *Dazed&Confused*, which ended up publishing them. She began to work regularly with the magazine and its online edition, *Dazed Digital*, documenting backstage action at fashion shows. In September 2011, she began covering the couture and ready-to-wear fashion weeks in London and Paris for *T: The New York Times Style Magazine*. She has also photographed haute couture shows in Paris for *AnOther* and had backstage images published in *V*, *L'Officiel* and British *Vogue*, among others. In addition, she has undertaken special commissions for Burberry and Mary Katrantzou, documented castings for various designers and made portraits for magazines such as *Apartamento*, German *Vogue* and British *Elle*.

Since her almost accidental entry into the world of professional fashion photography, Bobula has moved from strength to strength. Her aim is to carry on with the backstage shoots and other documentary-related projects. She has said that she sees herself less as a fashion photographer and more as a documentary photographer who often covers the fashion industry. She rarely does editorial work, explaining that this is 'probably because the way I work is almost the opposite of shooting editorials. There is no elaborate production and practically no planning involved.'

Despite this low-key approach, Bobula's work has managed to find its way into other platforms aside from magazines and websites. She has exhibited prints in Warsaw and London, and in 2011 her work was included in the limited-edition book *Holly and Kasia*, which was published by Ida Rhoda and featured images by Bobula and the British photographer Holly Hay.

Although she occasionally photographs still-life interior decors and architectural structures, most of Bobula's work is centred around the basic interaction between photographer and human subject and the idea of the chance encounter. Models are caught off-guard while being preened or dressed, or while waiting behind the scenes. Sometimes bored or laughing, they often engage directly with Bobula in a way that few other backstage photographers are able to elicit. Not one for elaborate set-ups, Bobula started out shooting on film with a Nikon FG-20, but more recently has switched to digital. She continues to work solely with the available light, arguing that 'you can have the most expensive equipment, but at the end of the day, it's all about the eye.'

We can see Bobula's keen but unobtrusive eye in the subtle gestures, elegant angles and quietly striking use of light in her modest yet beguiling compositions.

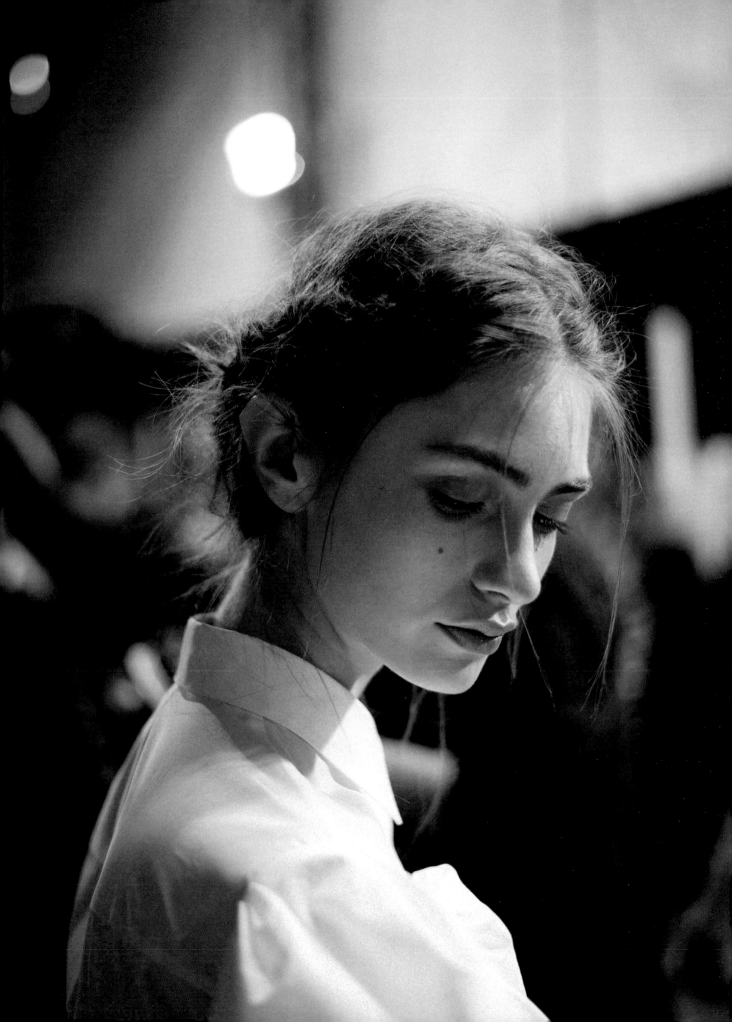

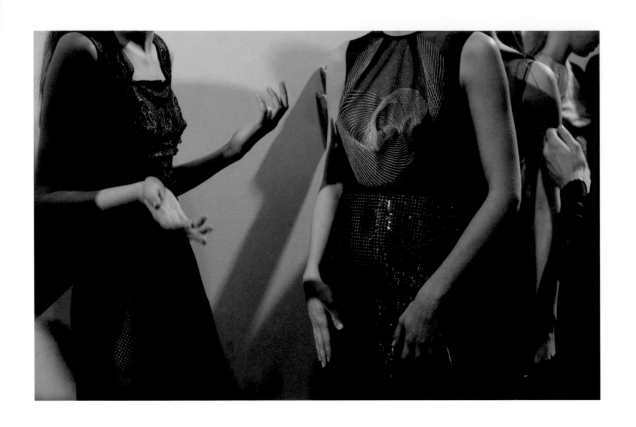

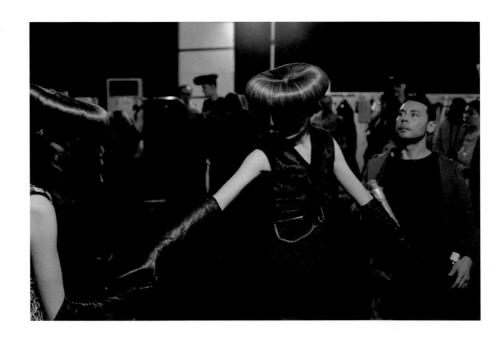

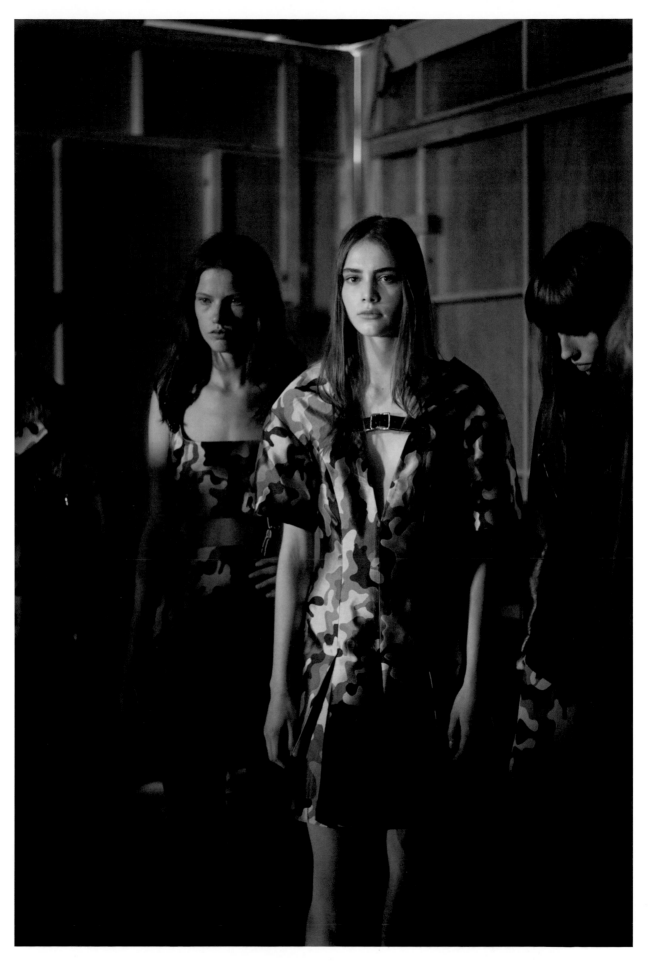

Kasia Bobula

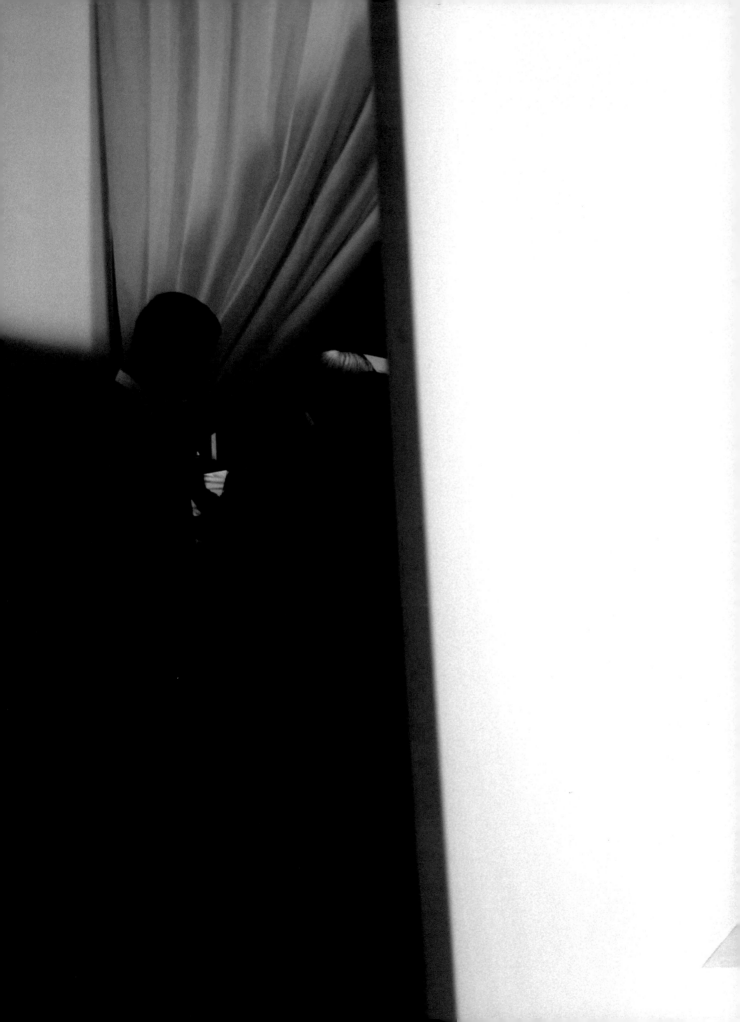

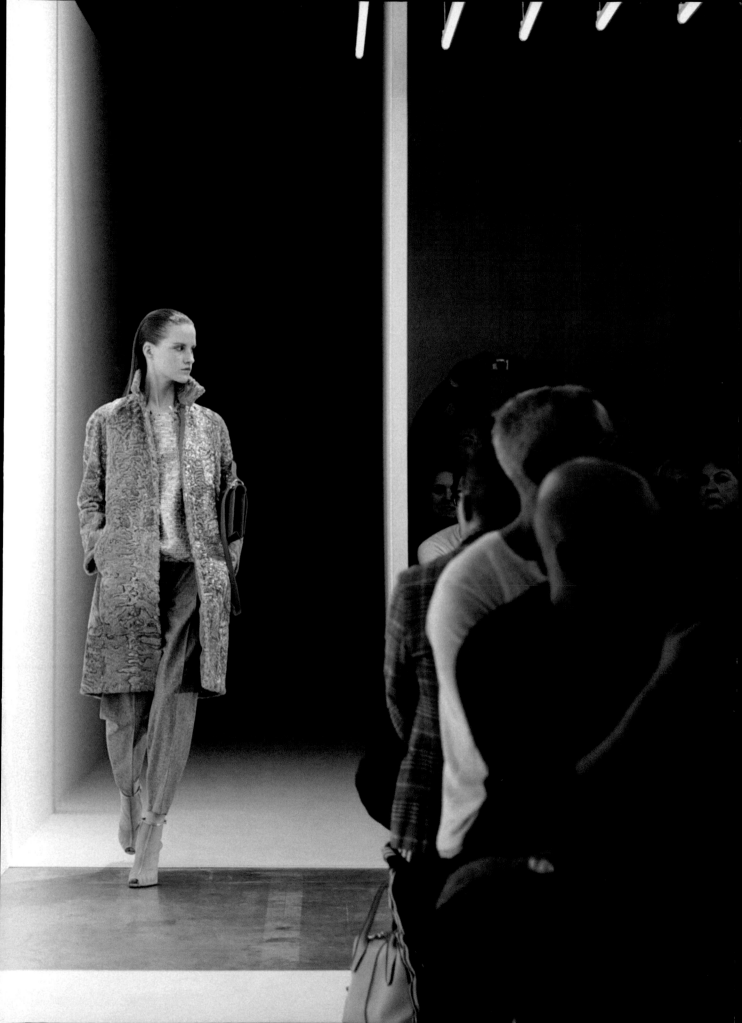

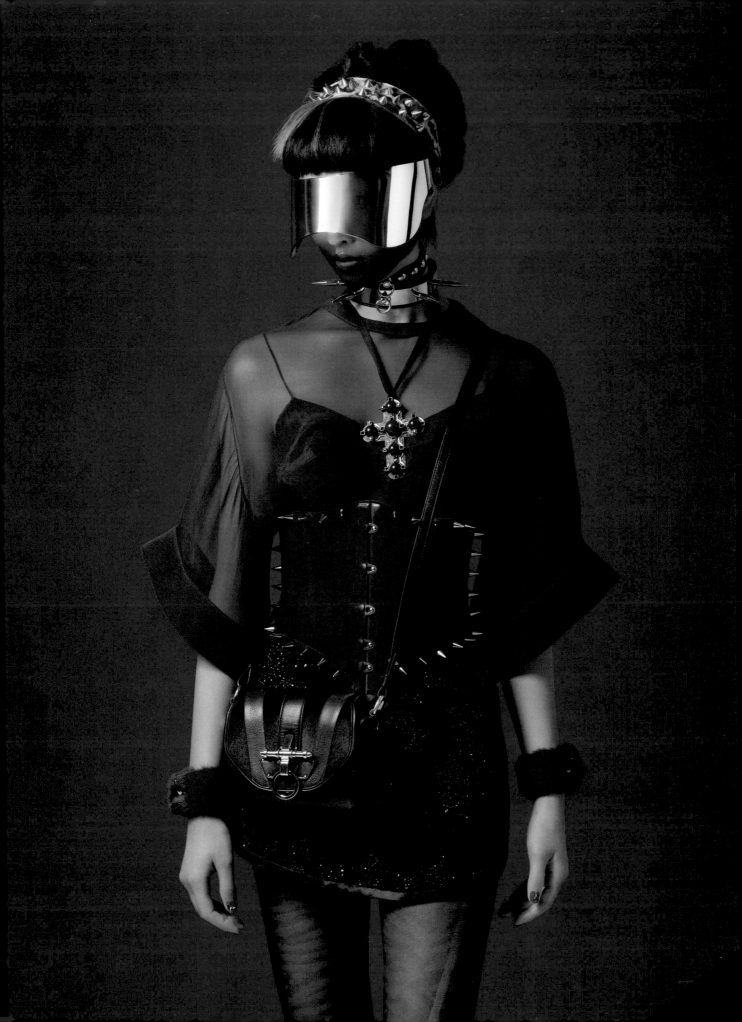

Timur Celikdag's photographs generate a sense of suspension, even isolation.

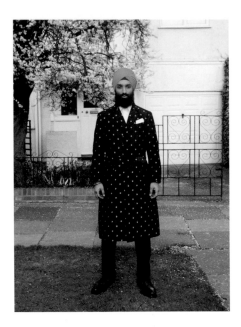

Born in a small working-class town in Germany to Turkish parents, Timur Celikdag (b. 1975) first began taking photographs around the age of 15 using a basic camera owned by his father. In order to pursue a career in photography, he moved to Hamburg to assist photographers and learn on the job. In 1999, he relocated to London to work with renowned German photographer Norbert Schoerner, remaining with Schoerner for two and a half years.

In 2003, Celikdag won the prestigious photography prize at the International Festival of Fashion and Photography in Hyères, France, for a series of male portraits shot on the streets of Istanbul. While in Hyères he met the founder and director of *i-D*, Terry Jones, an encounter that heralded the start of a successful working relationship with the iconic London-based magazine that continues to this day. Celikdag's first job for *i-D* was a portrait of the musical duo MU on London Bridge.

In addition to *i-D*, Celikdag's work has appeared in magazines such as *Fantastic Man, L'Uomo Vogue, Jalouse, Metal, Vogue Hommes International, Muse* and *GQ Style*. His photographs have been published in

books, including Terry Jones and Susie Rushton's *Fashion Now 2* (which was released by Taschen in 2008), and exhibited at various international locations: from Art Basel to the Chelsea Art Museum in New York and the Fashion and Textile Museum in London.

Winning the prize at Hyères and meeting Jones were catalysts for Celikdag's breakthrough into editorial, enabling him to pursue this path more closely after many years spent assisting. When asked what motivates him, he says: 'I never stop learning new things, and photography gets me into situations I wouldn't be experiencing otherwise.' This philosophy of discovery is visible in his photographs, which traverse fashion, portraiture, reportage and fine art. Images of people form the core of Celikdag's oeuvre, with subjects ranging from models and celebrities to strangers on the street. He enjoys the inherently unexpected and unpredictable nature of working with people; the fact that on a shoot 'whatever happens will differ from what I had imagined beforehand'.

These elements of chance, or chance encounters, that so captivate the photography sit in fascinating juxtaposition to the overall sense of calm evoked by his images. Whether shot in a studio or on location, Celikdag's photographs are restrained. They generate a sense of suspension, even isolation, an effect heightened by the photographer's ability to extract serene poses from his sitters and his very precise use of lighting. He rarely uses natural light as artificial light – anything from complicated photographic apparatus to street lamps and torches – allows him to play with the blurry line between the real and the 'not quite real'.

Celikdag is inspired by documentaries, films and books as well as by 'simply watching people on the street'. It is therefore unsurprising that he is partial to the work of some of the pioneers of street photography: Joel Meyerowitz, Lee Friedlander and Robert Frank, for example. His own work often makes tacit reference to the conventions of this tradition. Like much good street photography, Celikdag's images can be ambiguous: it is uncertain whether he has constructed the entire scenario or merely captured a fortuitous coincidence of light, setting and human presence.

36 'Banzai Gothique chez les Kawaii', *Libération Next*, 2012 — 38 'The Leading Man', *i-D*, 2012
39 'Towards Invisibility', *i-D*, 2004 — 40 'Zara', *i-D*, 2010 — 41 'Couleur Punk à l'Eau', *Libération Next*, 2012
42 'Do You Mind If We…Park…For A While?', *i-D*, 2010 — 43 'A Recital by Mr Konstantin Shamray', *Fantastic Man*, 2010

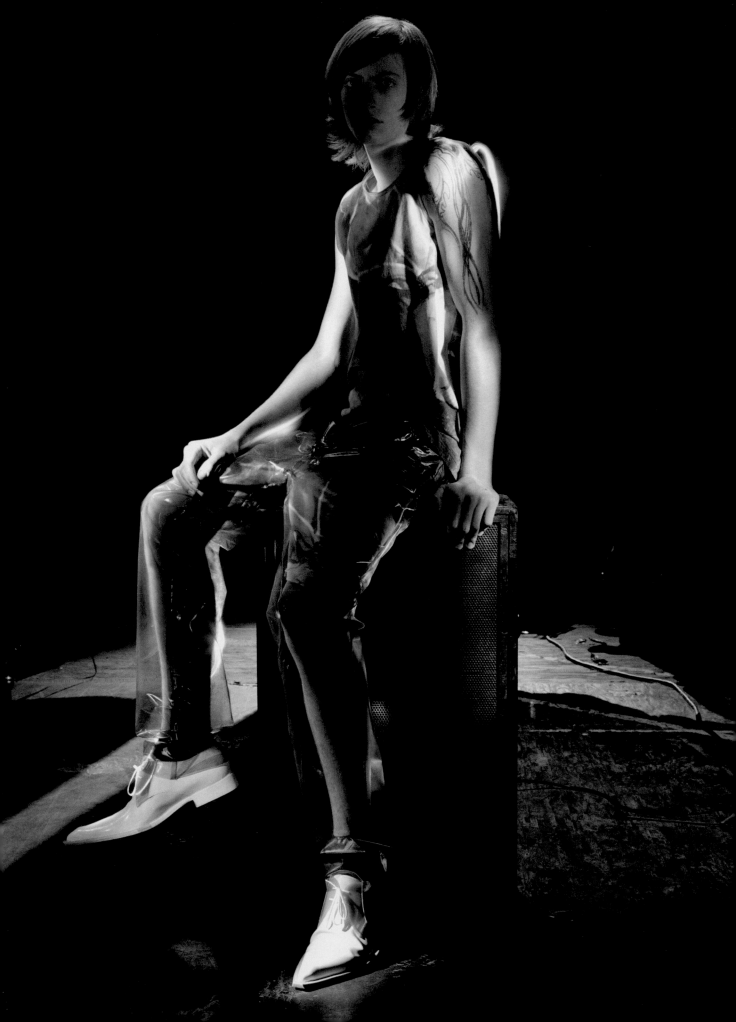

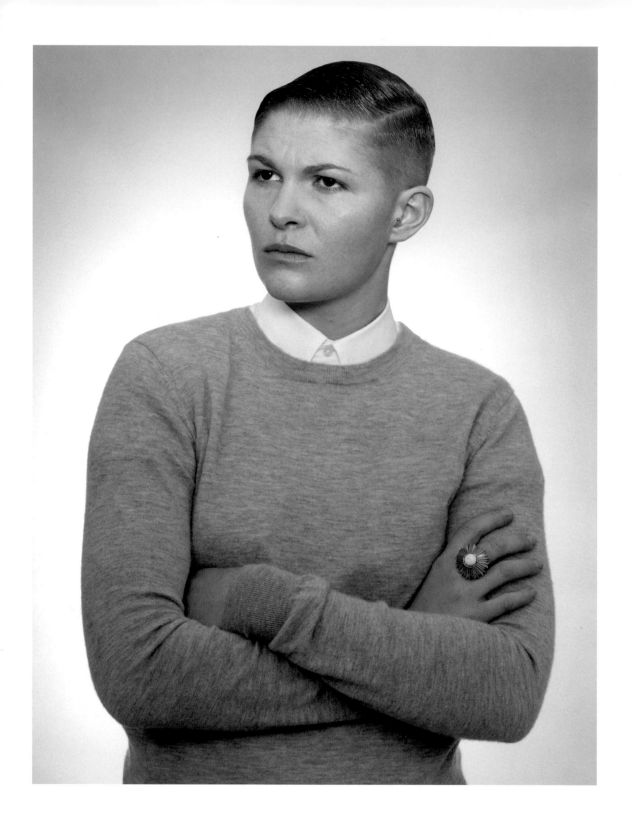

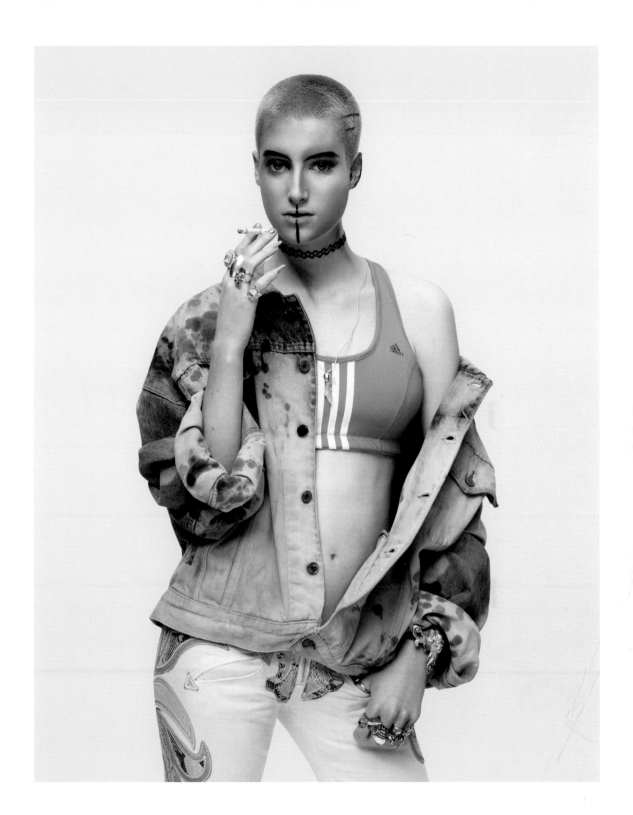

Timur Celikdag

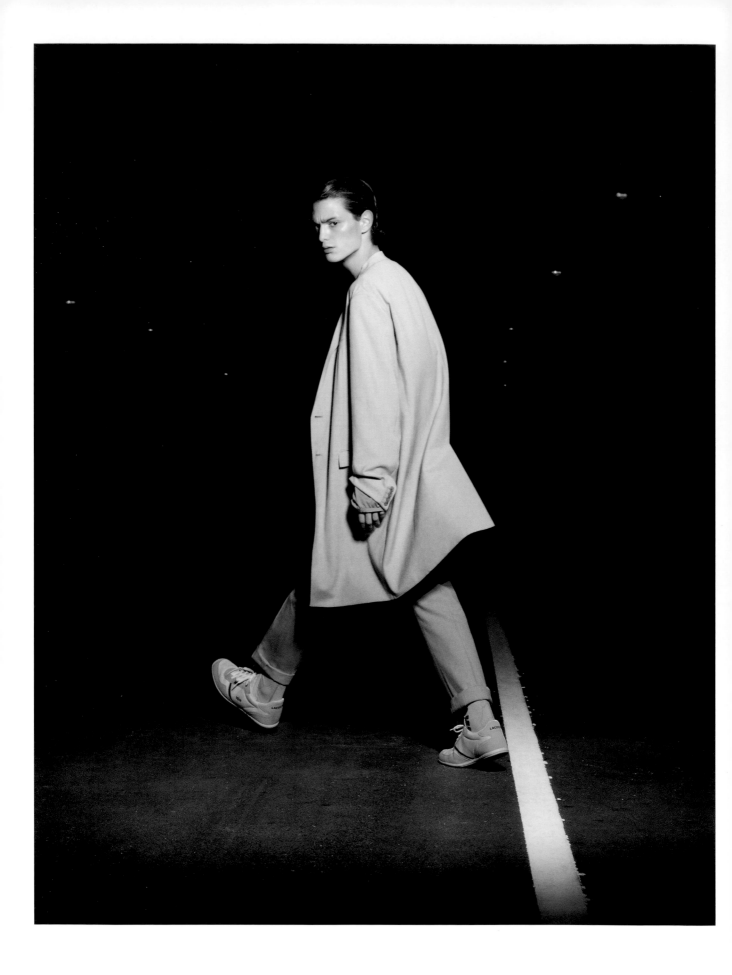

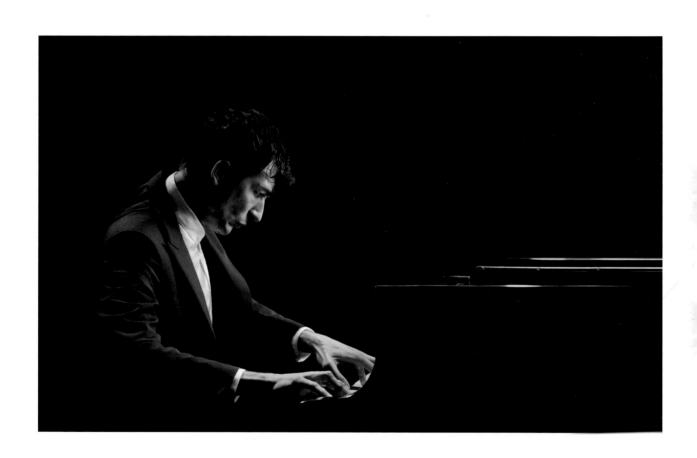

Timur Celikdag

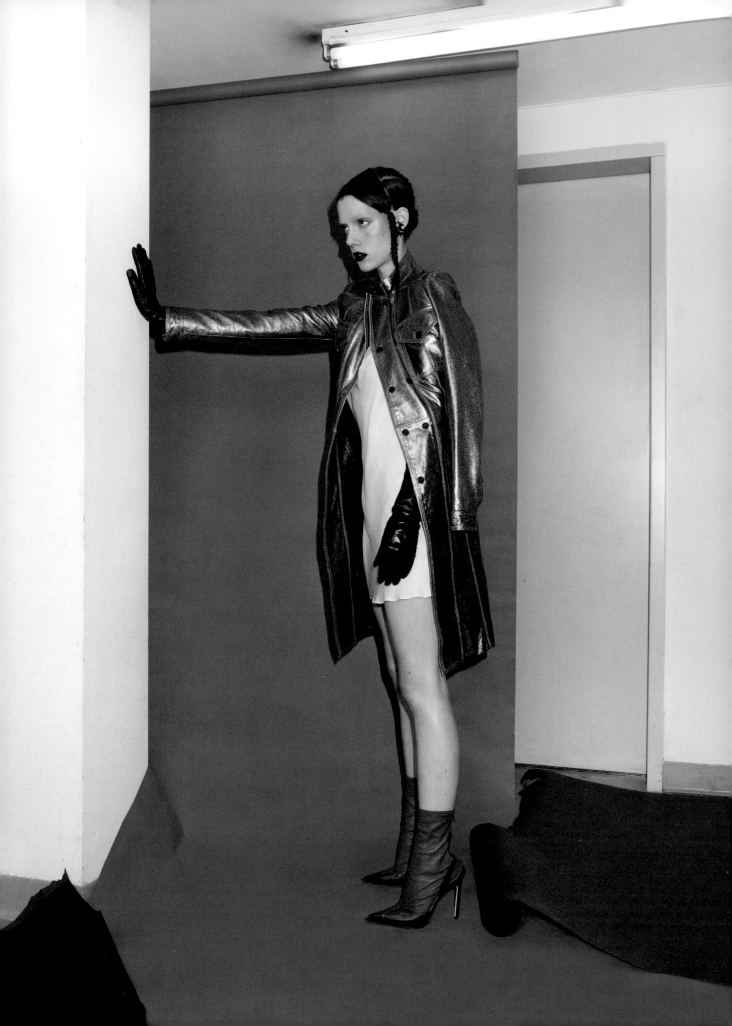

Charlie Engman is not afraid to playfully confront the artifice of his images.

Charlie Engman

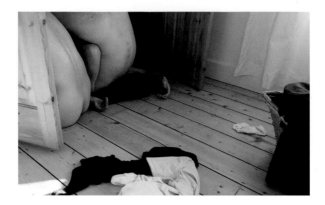

Originally from Chicago, Charlie Engman (b. 1987) lives and works in New York. He studied Japanese and Korean at the University of Oxford in the UK, graduating in 2009. Formerly a professional dancer and with an interest in performance and architectural sculpture, he combined his language degree with studies at the university's art department, the Ruskin School of Drawing and Fine Art. He began taking photographs as a means of making notes for his sculptural projects, notably creating *Domestic Diorama*, a series of abstract nudes or body studies often featuring himself as model, in 2008. These images were among his first attempts at using the camera to interrogate space, specifically the space of the photographic frame in relation to the human body and other sculptural forms. Engman posted the photographs on Flickr, where they caught the attention of *Dazed Digital*, which published them in 2009. After graduating, Engman worked as an assistant to New York-based designer Hillary Taymour of Collina Strada, creating lookbooks and advertising images. He collaborated with Taymour on his first published editorial, 'The End of Summer', an experiment in photocollage

for the September 2010 edition of *01* that combined portrait images with landscapes, abstract backgrounds and overlaid graphic components.

Though usually presented in sequence over a number of pages in a magazine layout, Engman's photographs could more accurately be thought of as singular images, rather than as components of a fashion story. They are in essence conceptual and visual solutions to the formal problem of picture-making that push the scope of what the photographer has to work with: clothes, models and props; studio sets or outdoors locations; light; and the potential of post-production. In each case, Engman responds to a slightly different question or set of preoccupations that is unique to the particular image and requires a specific approach and resolution. This non-linear process and presentation disrupts our conventional understanding of the way fashion images operate in magazine contexts.

Engman is not afraid to playfully and cleverly confront the artifice of his images. Time and again, the viewer is privy to the constructed nature of his workspace, where coloured paper backdrops, mirrored

surfaces, foam blocks, skylights, and door and window frames are used to build lo-fi temporary environments. These sets are often created by Engman himself as an integral part of the photographic process, although more recently he has enlisted the help of set designers.

One of Engman's most subversive yet beautiful editorials was 'Mom'. Published by Budapest-based biannual *The Room* in 2012, it featured his mother, Kathleen Engman, as model. By identifying his sitter as his 'Mom', Engman complicates his usually depersonalized approach where models are no more the subject of his photographs than the garments or other material components. In some images his mother is made up and styled, posing purposefully on set, but she also appears without makeup and nude except for a white banded collar in two head-and-shoulder portraits. Superbly styled by Tracey Nicholson, who often collaborates with Engman, the story poignantly confronts and debunks the ageism of the fashion industry. It continues Engman's exploration of vivid colour and space, simultaneously utilizing and exposing the illusion of infinite space implied by the rolled backdrop, a common studio prop.

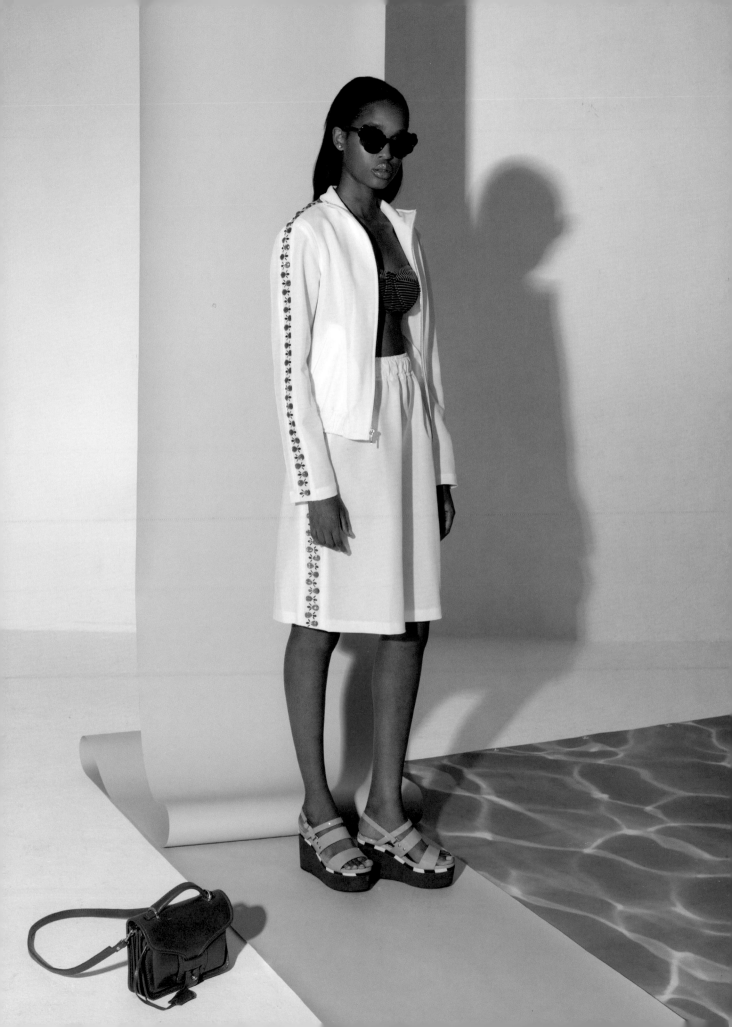

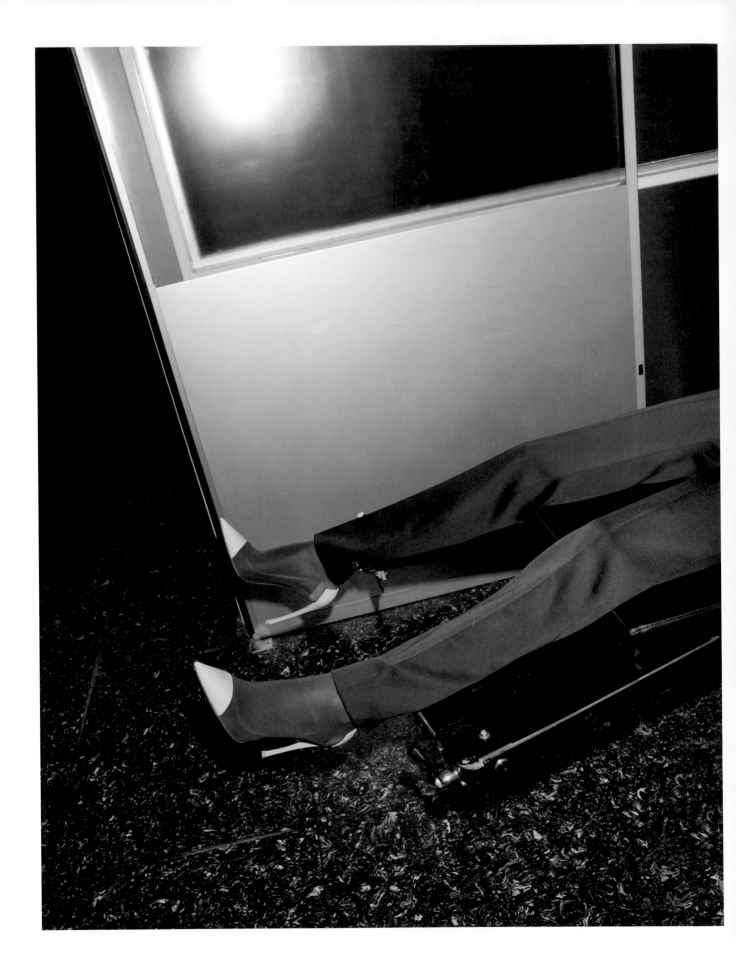

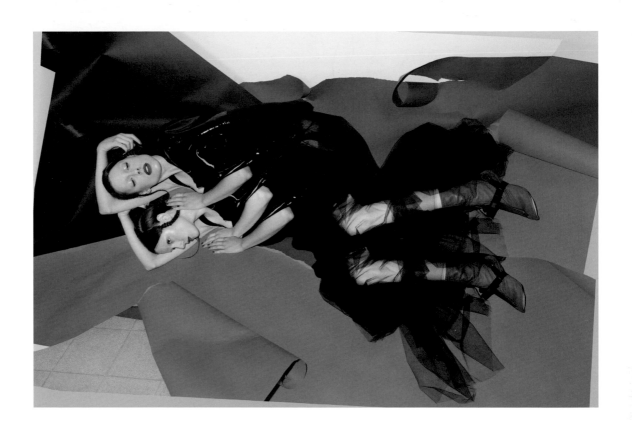

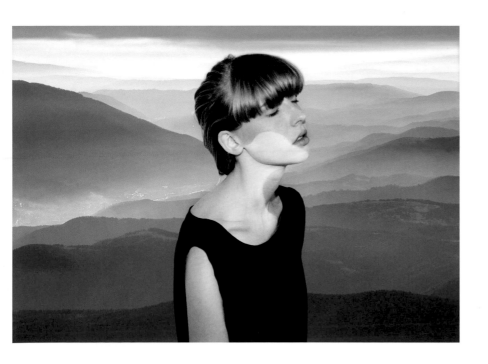

Charlie Engman

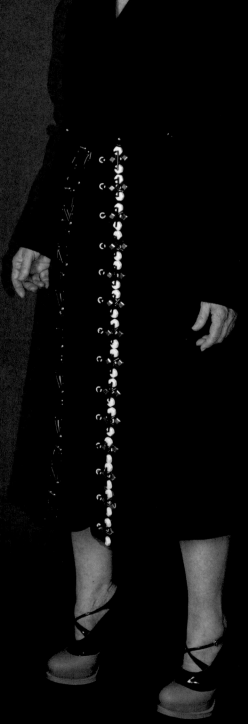

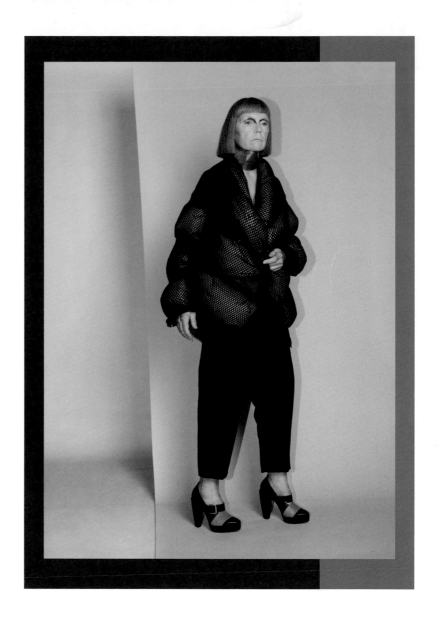

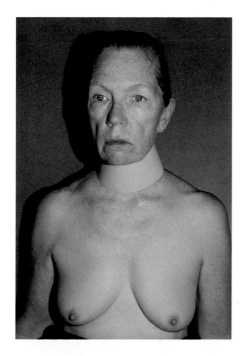

Charlie Engman

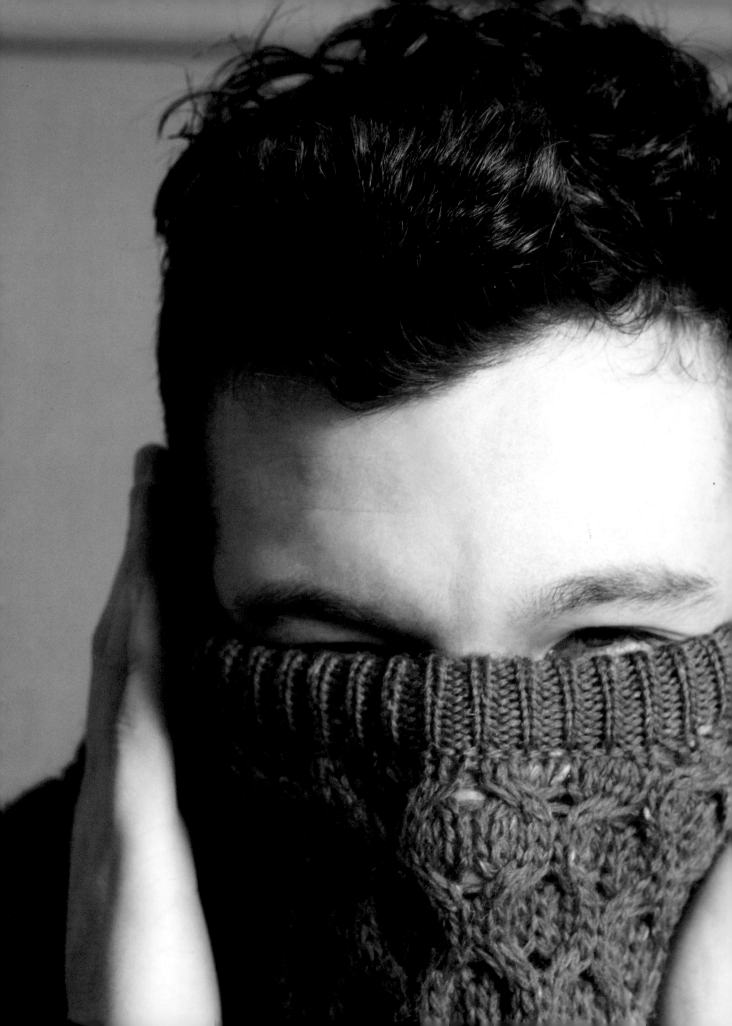

Jermaine Francis's images are remarkably consistent in style and purpose.

Jermaine Francis

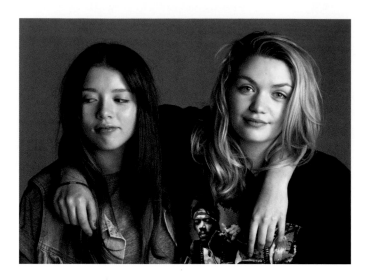

Jermaine Francis (b. 1974) lives and works in London. His interest in photography was sparked by the popular and counter culture of his teenage years: Roxy Music album covers and magazines such as *The Face,* which documented the British rave and dance music scene in the early 1990s. He graduated from Derbyshire University with a BA in photographic studies in 1997. After moving to London, he followed what was then the traditional route into fashion photography and began assisting, working with British portrait and fashion photographer Rankin and later at the offices of the fledgling *Dazed & Confused* magazine. The creative climate fostered in Francis a desire to develop his own personal vision and photographic language. This philosophy of honesty – of making photographs that are true to himself rather than adhering to fluctuating industry trends – was later reinforced during a period working for British photographer Corinne Day. It remains an important factor in the strength of his images.

It is not surprising, then, that since starting out on his own, Francis has not been inclined to follow the latest stylistic fads. His images are remarkably consistent in style with a clarity of purpose: he has a clean, classic approach to lighting and studio sets, as well as a highly personal engagement with his models that demonstrates a particular concern with conveying their unique personalities and styles. These characteristics are evident in an important lookbook made in 2011 for the Richard Nicoll shirt line 'Friends Utd', which featured apparently simple studio portraits, set against a draped backdrop.

Francis's stories are conceptualized as sequences rather than single static images, reflecting his belief that his subjects – be they models or celebrities – are multi-faceted. This approach was particularly convincing in a shoot with actor Nathan Stewart-Jarrett for David Bradshaw and Chris Bailey's menswear label Hunter Gather, as well as in a story for *Crash* with Susie Bick, and another for Net A Porter's

online magazine, *The Edit,* with legendary model Penelope Tree.

Stylistically, over the course of his career, Francis has progressed towards an increasingly effortless quality of fluidity through a nuancing of gesture and pose. Particularly in the transition from analogue to digital, which he has embraced with seamless sophistication, he has pursued and achieved a refinement and balance of in-shot lighting, with less synthetic post-production than many of his contemporaries working in the studio.

A frequent contributor to *Crash* magazine, which has been an important supporter and commissioner of his work, Francis has also produced editorials for *Tank, Twin, The Sunday Times Style,* and Russian and Chinese *Vogue.* His commercial clients include Gieves & Hawkes, Mr Porter, Roksanda Ilincic, ME + EM and Wrangler.

52 'Callum' for Hunter Gather, 2012 — 54 'Rae and Dora' from 'The Girls Next Door', *Test Mag*
55 'Nathan' for Hunter Gather, 2012 — 56 **above** Susie Bick, *Crash,* 2011
56 **below** Penelope Tree, *The Edit,* 2013 — 57 'Jamie' for Richard Nicoll 'Friends Utd', 2011

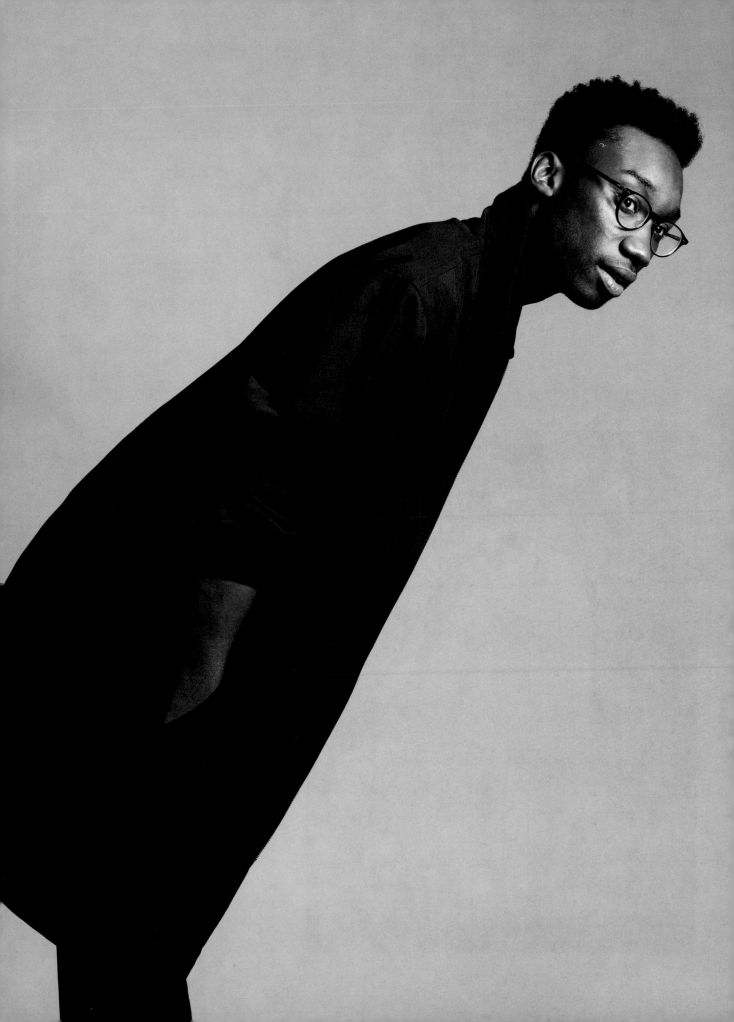

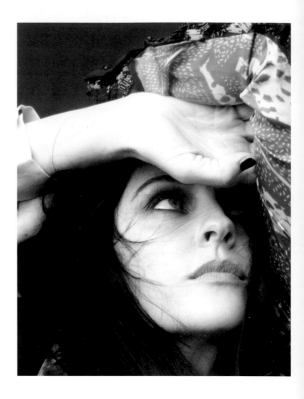

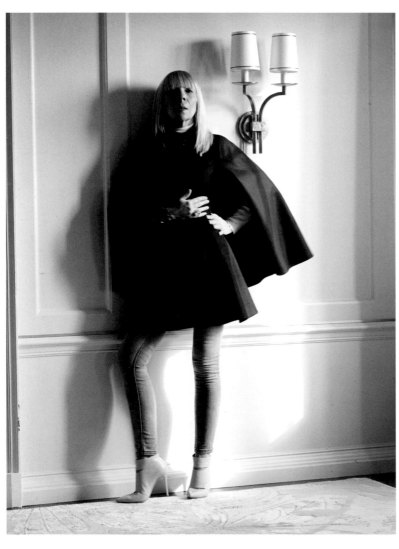

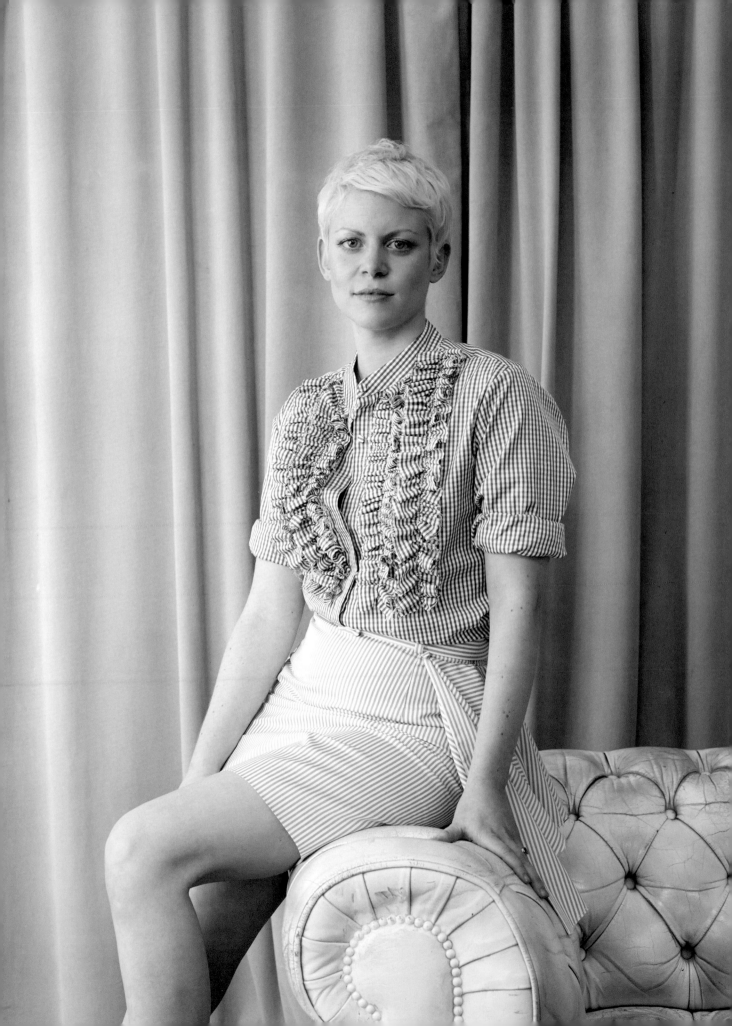

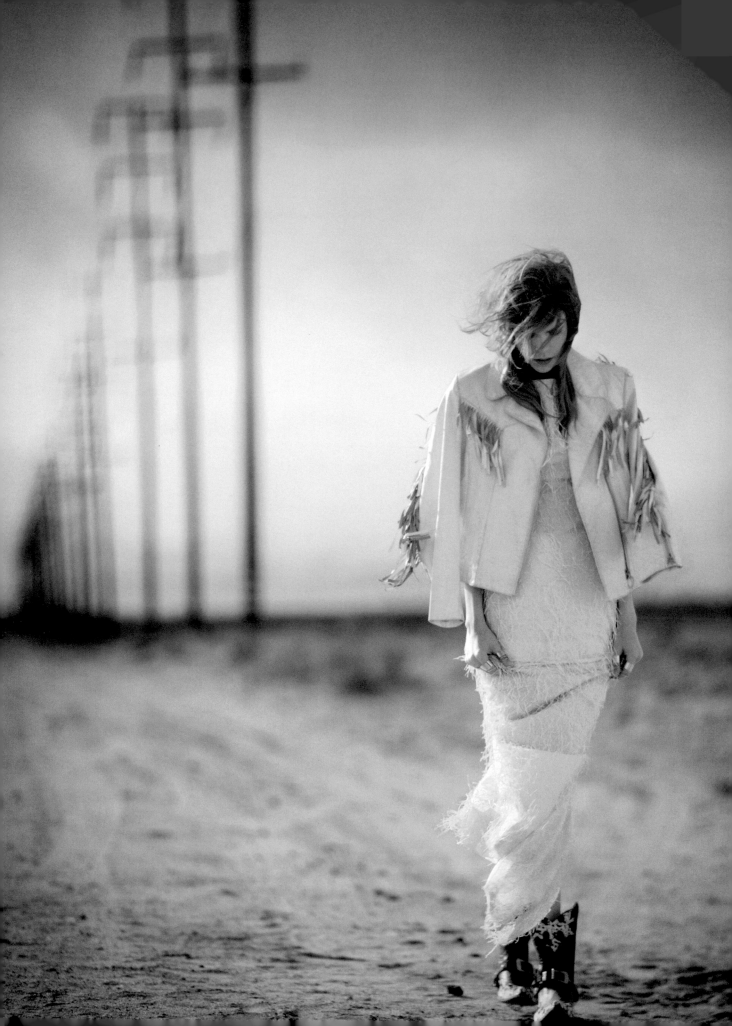

Boo George's photographs are at once epic and intimate, romantic and tough.

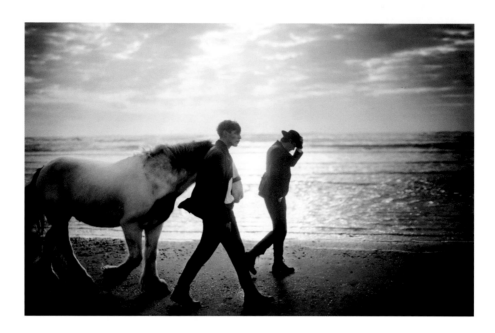

Born in County Wicklow, Ireland, Boo George (b. 1981) studied media in Dublin before moving to Middlesbrough, north-east England, to study photography at Cleveland College of Art and Design. After graduating in 2004 he relocated to London, where he worked for British photographers Julian Broad (who started out as an assistant to Lord Snowdon) and Phil Poynter. His first editorial was published in *i-D* magazine in 2008. Two years later, after making a series of striking black-and-white portraits of Zambian diamond miners for the creative agency Saturday, he received a commission from the editor of *Love*, Katie Grand, for whom he continues to work.

Over the next few years, George's editorial credits amassed to include *Vogue*, *Teen Vogue*, *L'Uomo Vogue*, *Numéro Homme*, *Arena Homme +* and *Twin*. He has also worked for a range of commercial clients, such as Topman, Aquascutum, Hardy Amies, Bergdorf Goodman and Joseph. In 2013 he was the winner of 'The Shot', a prestigious talent search run by *W* magazine and the International Center of Photography.

George's photographs, which are taken on location, are at once epic and intimate, romantic and tough. They are often inhabited by misfits, bohemians, dissidents and wanderers, characters of the photographer's own making that mix references to popular culture with allusions to film and music. His male and female subjects possess an unusual beauty and exude a sense of youthful rebellion. Fashion garments are an important element in the storytelling, and the gap-tooth or shaven-headed models George favours are more likely to convey an attitude through an expression or a gesture rather than a formal pose. In the best of his work, these anti-heroes and heroines have a certain depth and conviction that invites us to imagine them beyond the still image, imbuing the photographs with a feeling of restless movement.

An interesting point of reference could be the now classic fashion photographs taken in the 1980s and '90s by German photographer and filmmaker Peter Lindbergh. George's photographs reinterpret Lindbergh's glamour while also descending from early twentieth-century studio photography, Hollywood screen icons and the documentary tradition. Although George works digitally, he is much more interested in getting a shot in-camera than during post-production. He has frequently spoken of his admiration for Richard Avedon, the great twentieth-century American photographer. Like Avedon, who was famed for his masterful ability to incisively frame his subjects and his precision and directness in making portraits, George looks for something particular in each of his sitters. His stories are embedded in their locations, with the photographer then engaging his models in pursuit of the right shot, using the capacity of digital image capture to edit on set. His work is a rare combination of imaginative narrative, documentary-style composition and an intuitive awareness of the importance of timing and pose.

58 *i-D*, 2013 — **60** 'Nomades', *Numéro Homme*, 2012 — **61** Agyness Deyn, *Love*, 2010
62 above 'Camel & Neutrals / Modern Classics', *Arena Homme +*, 2010 — **62 below** Dree Hemingway, *Love*, 2010
63 left *i-D*, 2012 — **63 right** *Twin*, 2009 — **64–65** 'Cirque du Chic: Young Hollywood', *Teen Vogue*, 2012

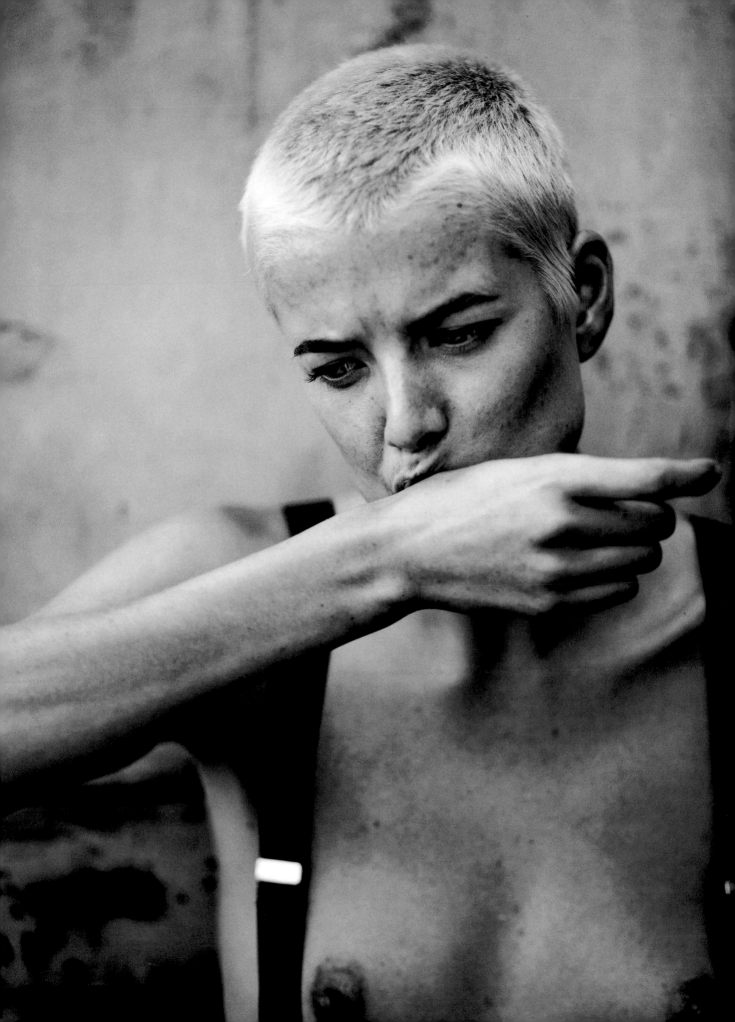

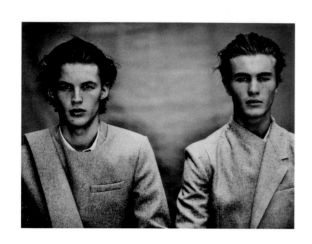

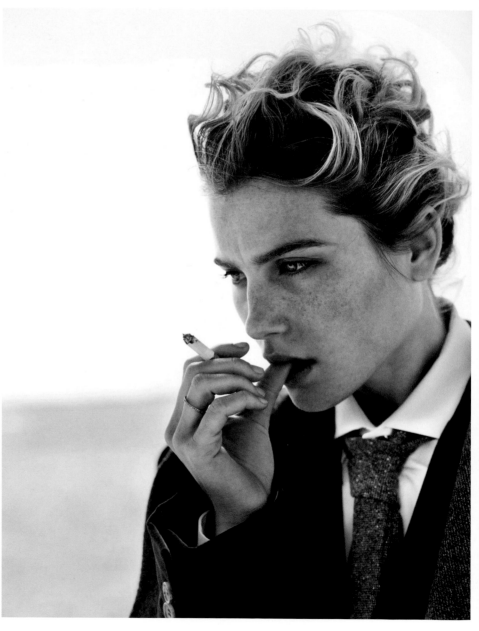

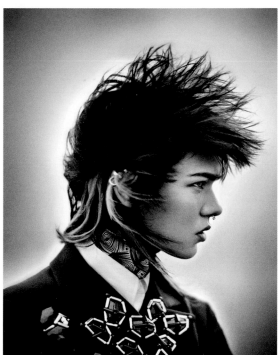

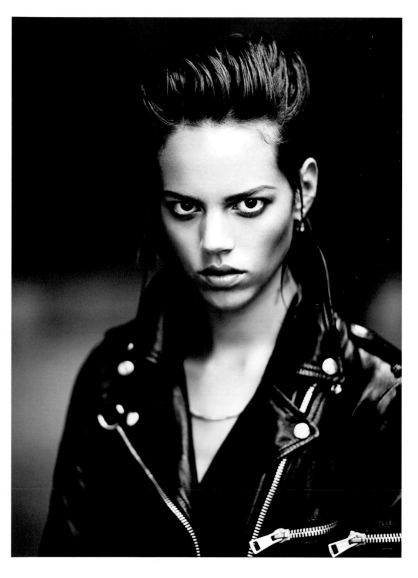

Boo George

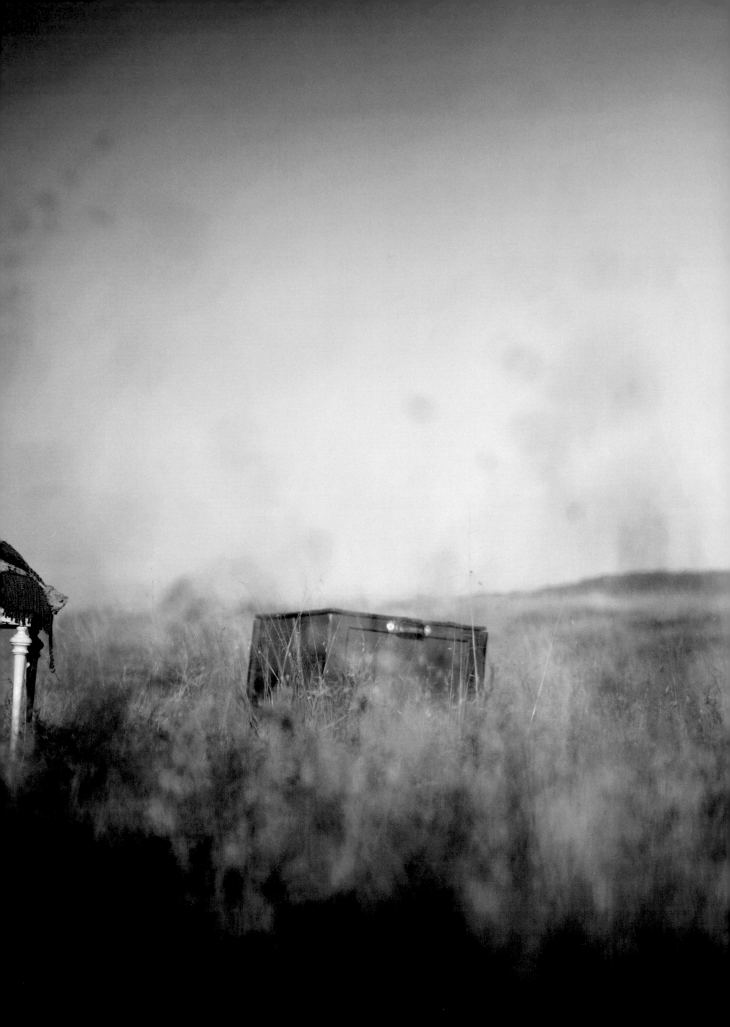

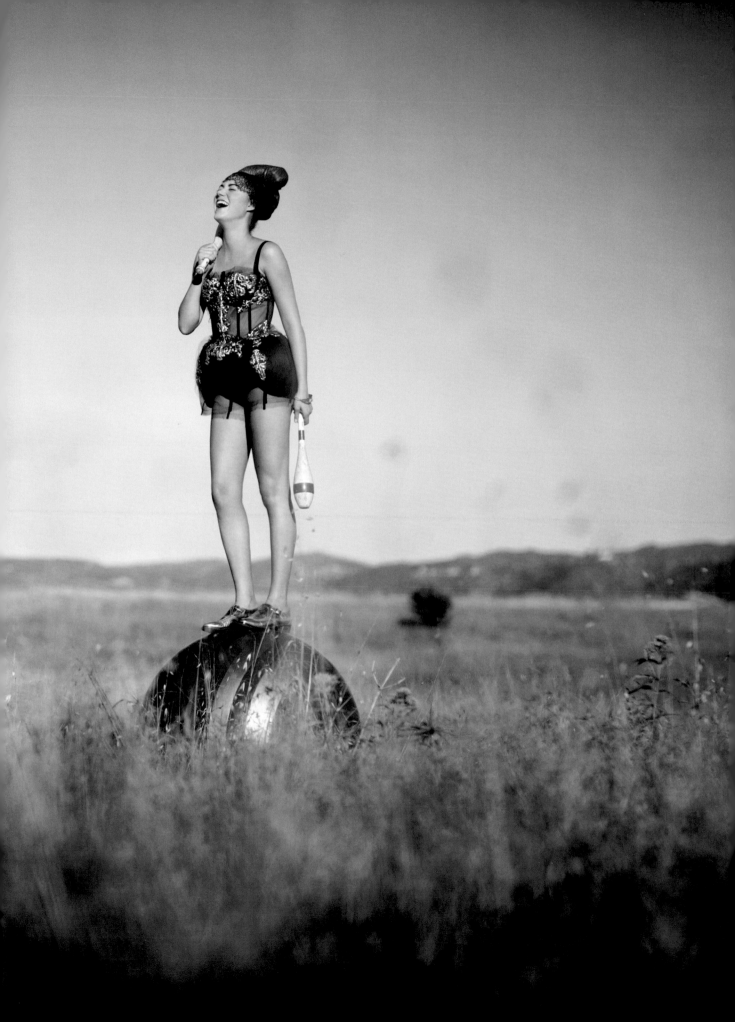

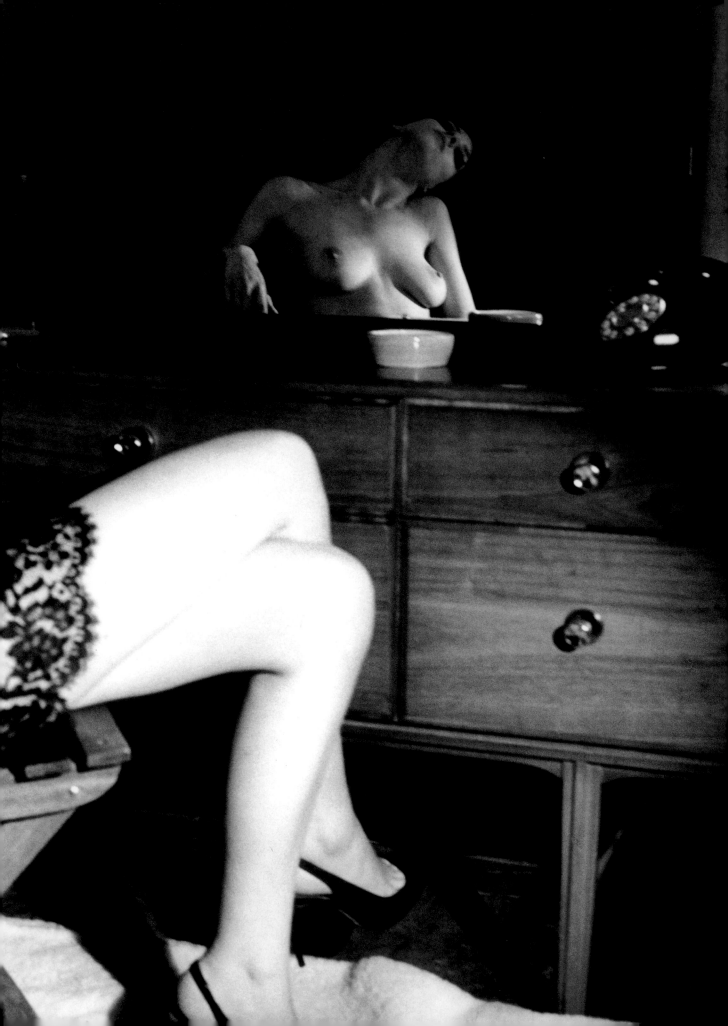

Jonathan Hallam's use of film is evident in the rich colours and tonal range of his photographs.

Jonathan Hallam

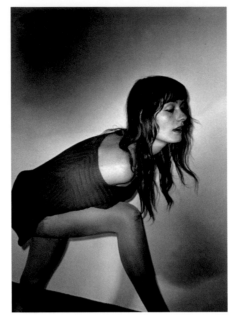

The career of British photographer Jonathan Hallam (b. 1972) began largely unwittingly via his work as a hairdresser. He began cutting hair at the age of 15 and eventually came to work as a session stylist for some of the industry's top creatives, including stylists Marie-Amélie Sauvé and Jane How, and photographers Paolo Roversi, Satoshi Saïkusa, and Mert and Marcus. Known during this time as Jonny Drill, Hallam gained a reputation for his brutal and angry haircuts and his forward-thinking approach to hairstyling. He often made hairpieces out of unusual materials such as denim and fur, for instance, or shaved large chunks out of models' hair well before the half-shaved look was on trend (and much to the dismay of the girls' agents). This ostensibly aggressive attitude masked a much more subtle interest in form and a desire to push the boundaries of contemporary fashion imagery. It was less a conscious tactic of gaining a rebel reputation and more a way of existing in and confronting a world that seemed very prescribed. Unsurprisingly, Hallam's approach to photography is very similar.

While assisting British hairstylist Eugene Souleiman in the late 1990s at Maison Martin Margiela shows, Hallam took backstage photographs with a disposable camera. He moved to Paris in 1999 and by the following year was working with Margiela as an official backstage photographer while also creating lookbooks and shooting in-store images for the Belgian designer. Hallam's Paris work includes many avant-garde shoots, often collaborations with stylist Roxane Danset, as well as portraits of friends and neighbours, and documentation of his life in the city. His photographs from this period are usually black and white, and often hand-printed, a technique with which he has continued to experiment throughout his career.

The freedom of Hallam's time in Paris means that the line between his personal and professional work from this period is often blurry. His collaboration with Margiela led to an association with *Purple* magazine that continues to this day. Since returning to London in 2006, Hallam has worked as a freelance photographer for many progressive fashion publications, including *10*, *Under/Current*, *French*, *Sleek*, *Zoo*, *Dazed & Confused*, *Dossier*, *Plastique*, *Ponytail*, Turkish *Vogue* and *Self Service*.

At the start of his photographic career, Hallam always shot on film, somehow managing to resist the mandates of an industry with an almost exclusively digital commercial sector. His use of film is evident in the deep quality, rich colours and tonal range of his photographs, as well as in the light leaks and visible film perforations that embrace imperfection.

Recently, however, Hallam has become more open to the idea of shooting digitally and he now employs the technology without losing any of his signature quirkiness. While there is a more subdued quality to his digital work, the key stylistic elements are not lost. Editing remains minimal and, crucially, he continues to photograph his subjects in poses that are unexpected and even awkward. Captured seemingly in-between shots, Hallam's models appear to be lost in themselves or engrossed in posing for the camera, a disposition that is often enhanced by additional lighting or mirrors and other reflective surfaces. These props are not used self-reflexively to reveal the photographer at a remove from his subjects; instead, they reinforce the models' presence while subtly reminding us of the ultimate inability of photography to capture someone wholly.

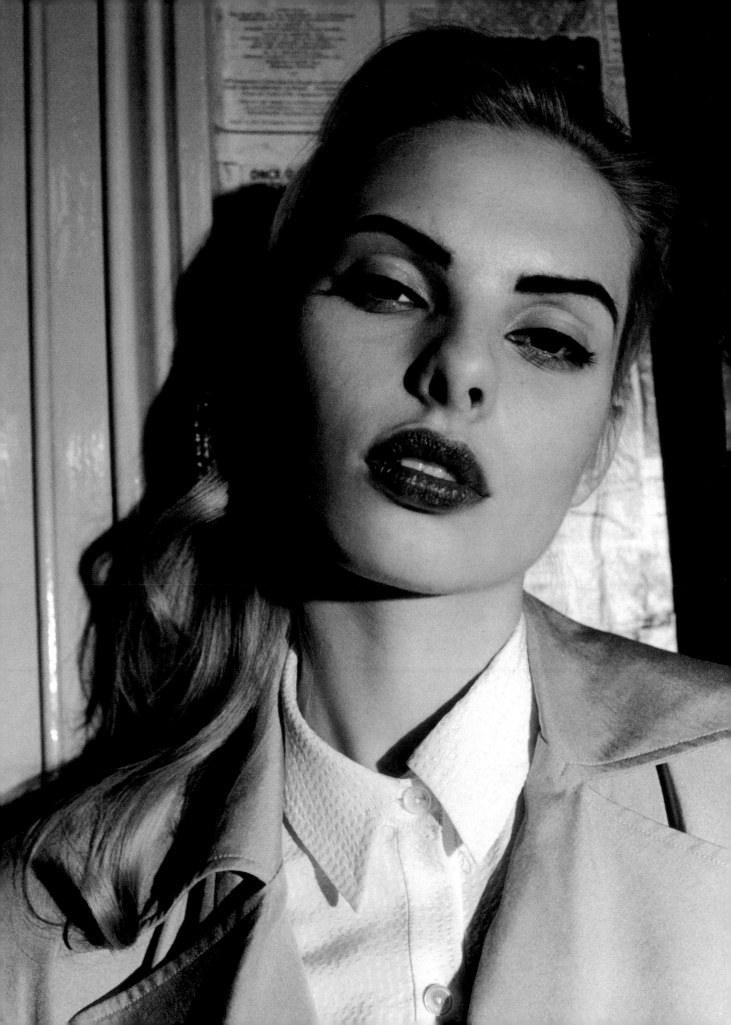

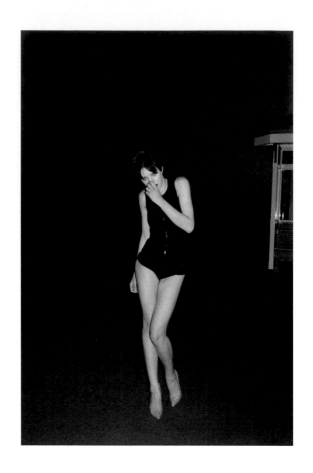

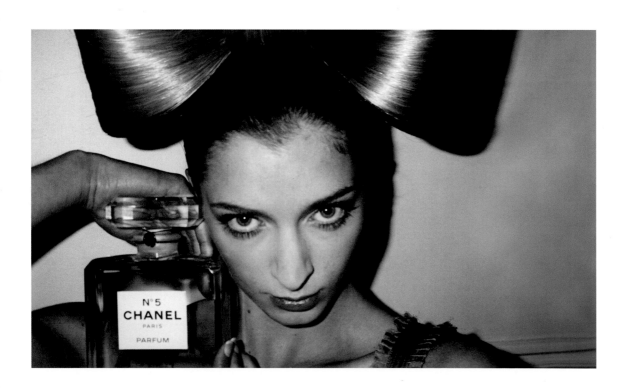

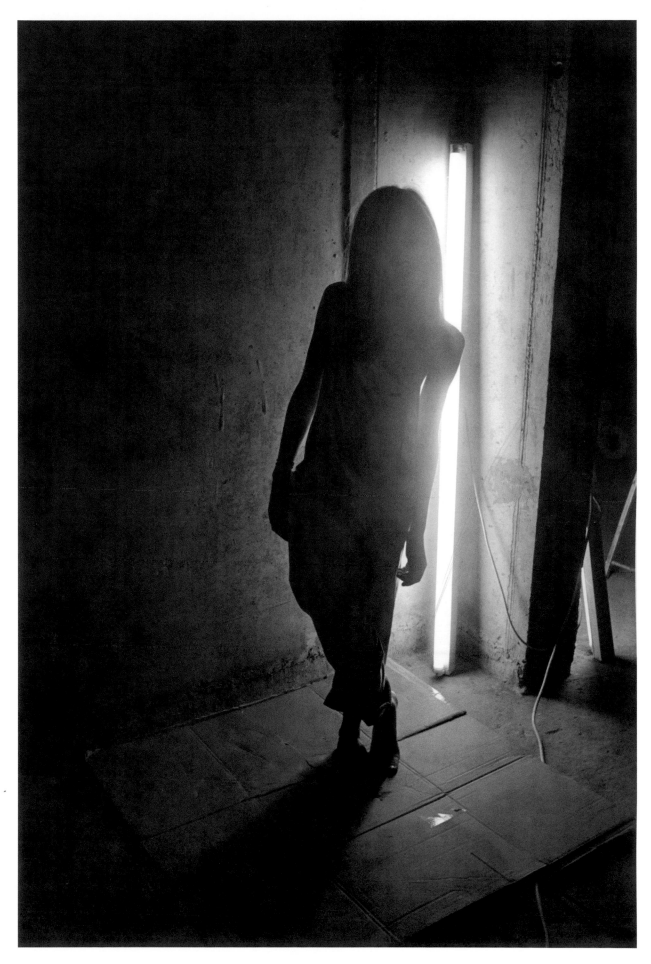

Jonathan Hallam

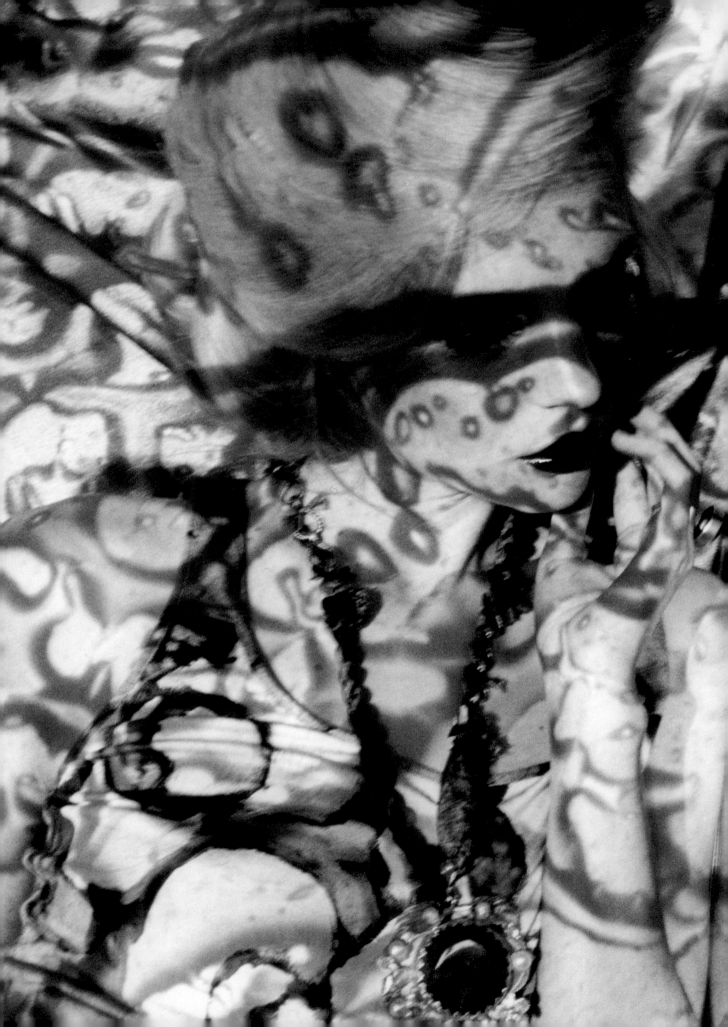

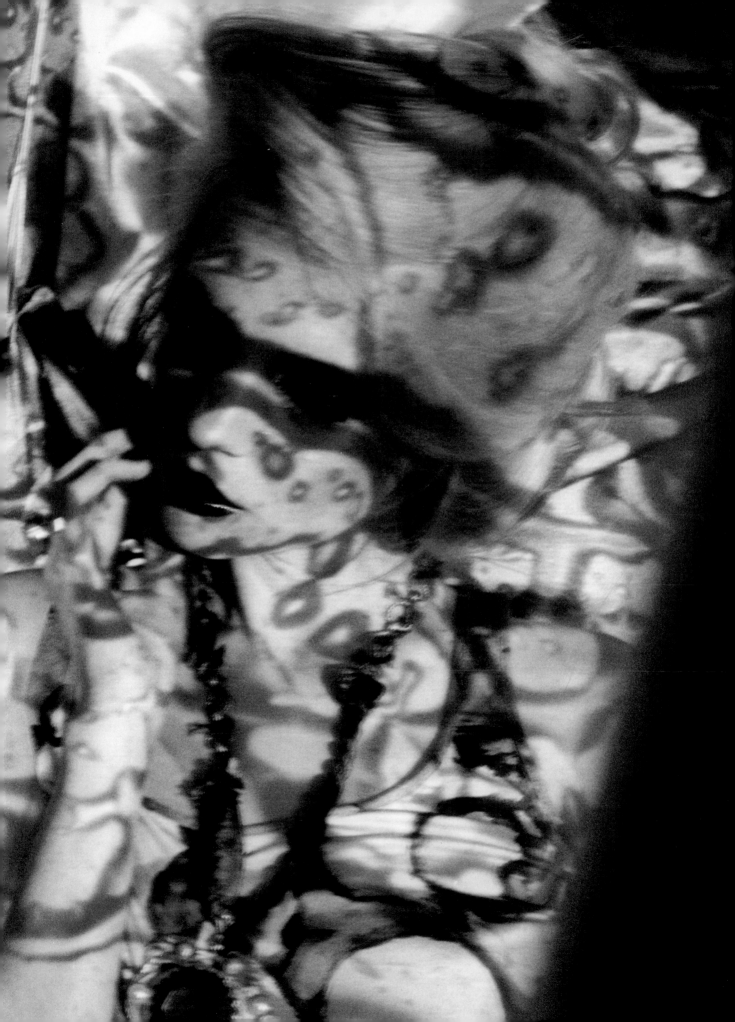

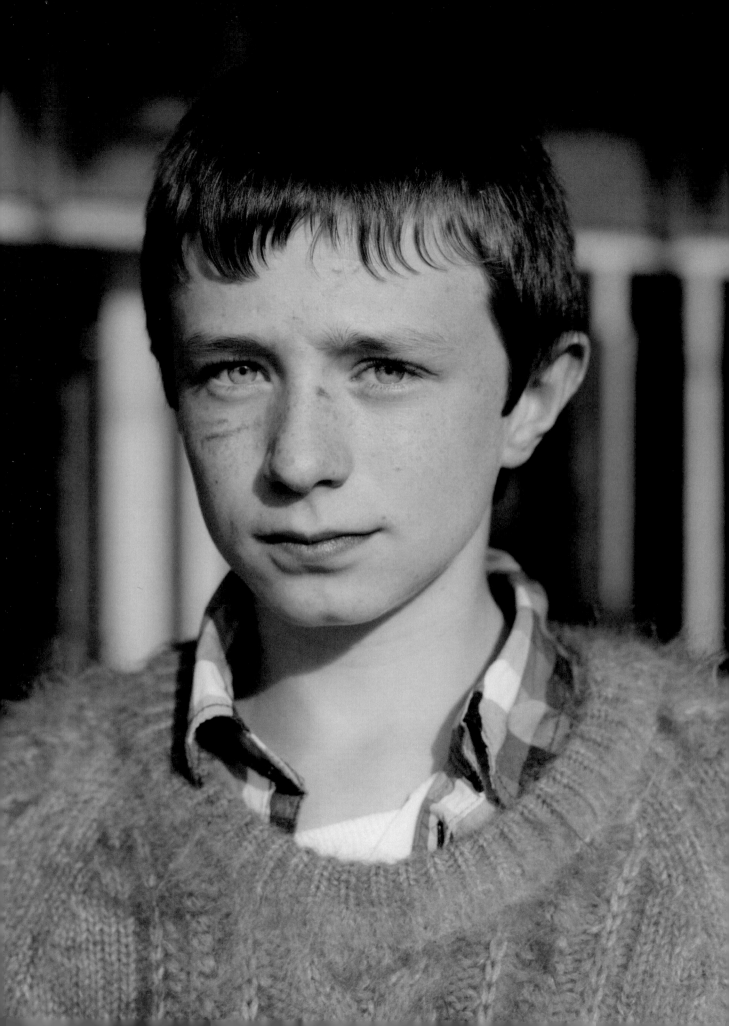

Jamie Hawkesworth moves easily between documentary, portrait and fashion photography.

Jamie Hawkesworth

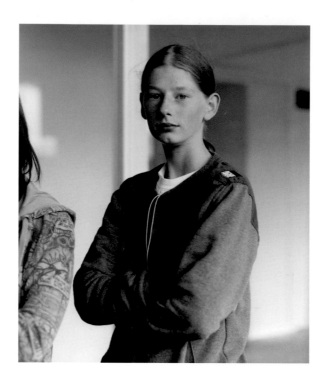

Jamie Hawkesworth (b. 1987) is a British photographer who lives in London. In 2010, shortly after graduating from the University of Central Lancashire in Preston, north-west England, with a BA in photography, he produced a startlingly beautiful breakthrough work in collaboration with artists Adam Murray and Robert Parkinson: the self-published, limited-edition folio *Preston Bus Station*. Hawkesworth's images of young people at an old bus station earmarked for demolition were the basis on which he received his first editorial commission for *Dazed & Confused*. In their balance between formality and empathetic sensitivity, the colour photographs of individual teenagers relate to the influential portrait series of Dutch photographer Rineke Dijkstra and British photographer Nigel Shafran, while also continuing a strand of British social documentary centred around the youth culture and class politics of a particular region or place. Hawkesworth met his subjects by chance – they were not cast or styled – and he displays in this self-initiated project an easy movement between documentary, portrait and fashion photography.

There is largely no self-conscious tension between Hawkesworth's personal and commissioned work as he approaches the two sides of his practice with the same processes in search of a similar aesthetic. So, for example, in a 2010 editorial for *The New British* magazine, he travelled with stylist Victoria Young to South Shields, near Newcastle. Like *Preston Bus Station*, the story was street cast and comprises a sequence of photographs of solitary teenagers at the seaside, in the town centre or in suburban gardens. While in some images these subjects appear to be unstyled and caught unawares, at other times Young intervenes, layering purposefully oversized and often incongruous high-fashion garments with the teenagers' own clothes.

For another, ongoing series of portraits Hawkesworth has travelled across the UK by train, taking photographs of unstyled young people with a medium-format film camera. Here, fashion – not only his subjects' overall style, but also the details of their outfits and the way they wear their clothes – is of fundamental importance to the portraits. Although they were not made for magazine publication, the images reference the language of fashion photography as the subjects pose like models. Hawkesworth constructs stories like fashion editorials, with portrait photographs punctuated by landscapes, cityscapes or shots of local landmarks.

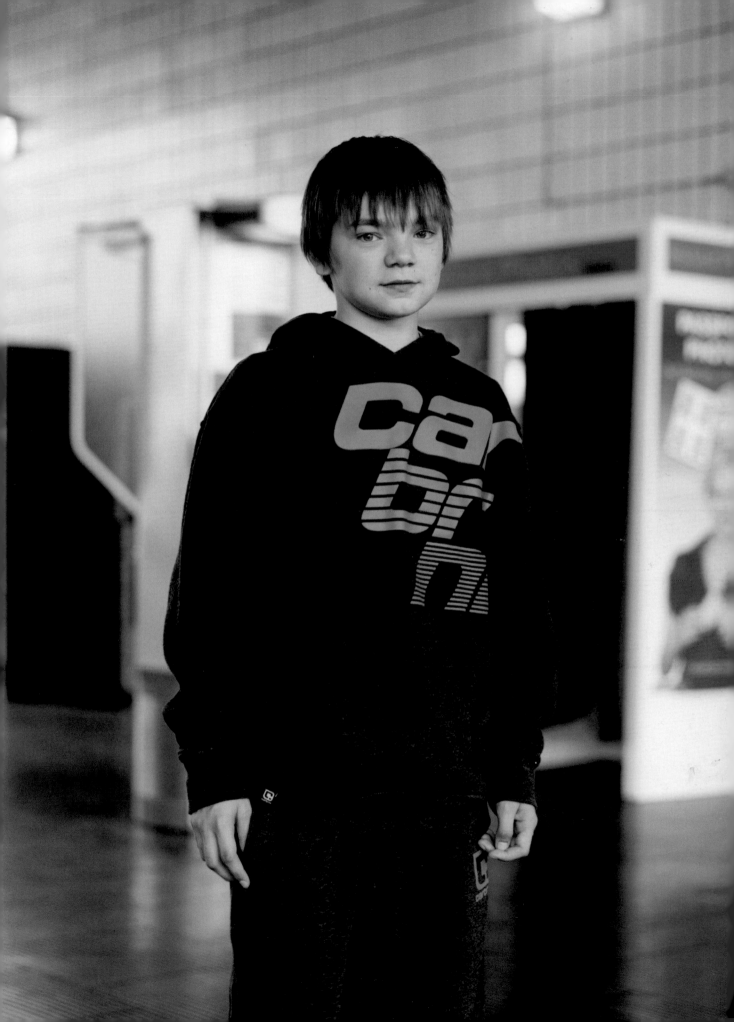

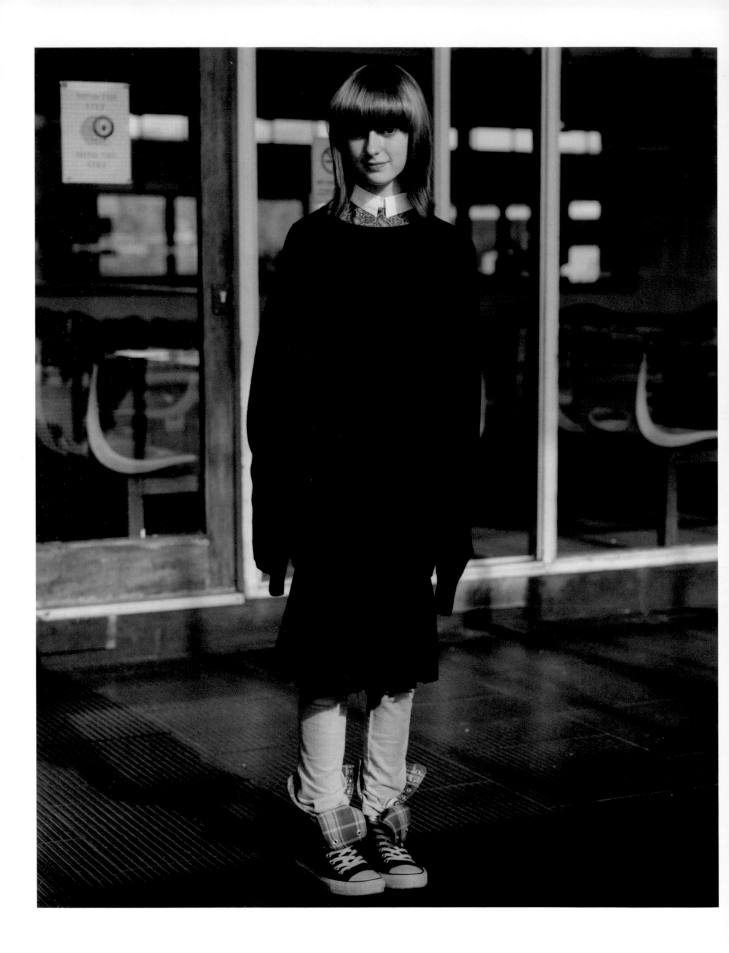

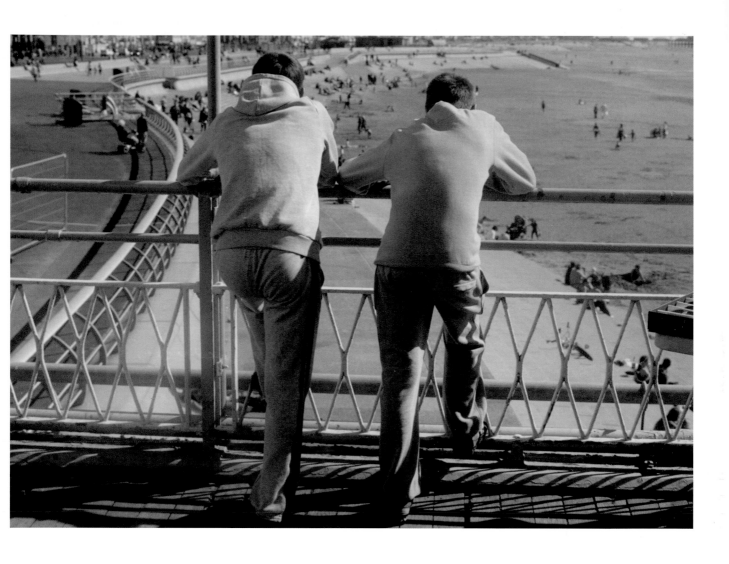

Jamie Hawkesworth

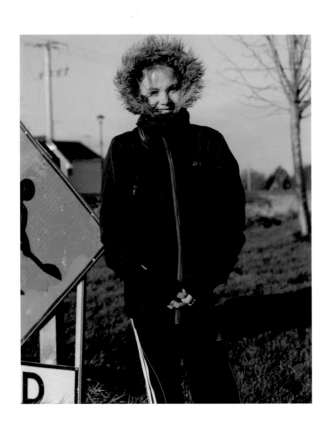

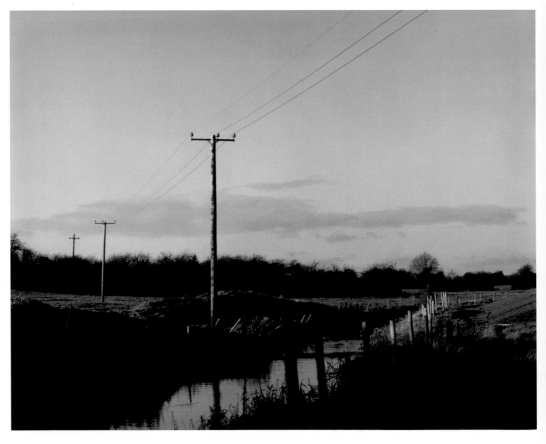

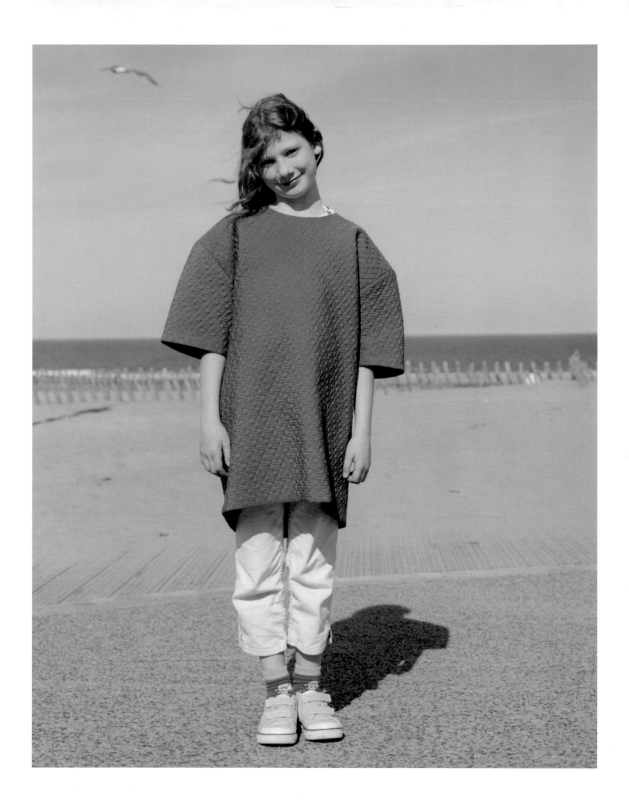

Jamie Hawkesworth

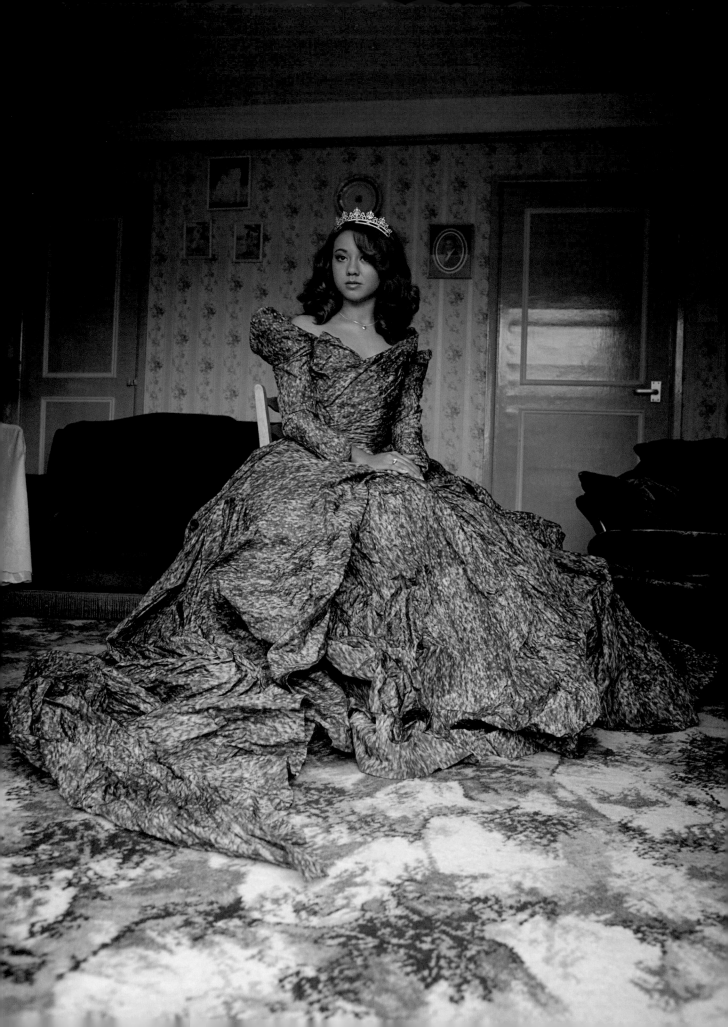

Alice Hawkins allows her sitters to revel in their personal style and celebrate their individuality.

Alice Hawkins

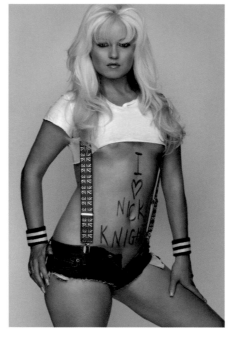

Alice Hawkins (b. 1979) is a British photographer based in London. She graduated from Camberwell College of Arts in 2002 with a degree show featuring photographs of a party she threw for an eclectic group of friends. Not long after finishing university, she was commissioned by *i-D* magazine to cover the London party scene. Hawkins was a finalist in *The Independent* /American Express Fashion Photography Competition in 2003, the year the judging panel included designer Alexander McQueen and photographer Nick Knight, who became her mentor. In an early self-portrait from 2007, she posed as an all-British Page Three girl with 'I ♥ Nick Knight' scrawled in red lipstick across her bare stomach. This image anticipates many of the hallmarks of her photographic practice, such as the importance of dress up, performance and sexual fantasy.

One strand of Hawkins's editorial work revolves around her series of stylized 'fashion portraits' celebrating female beauty outside of mainstream or high-fashion contexts: photographs populated with Page Three girls, Japanese women dressed as maids, original Playboy Bunnies and East Anglian beauty pageant hopefuls. For other projects, she has photographed men and women encountered on road trips across the USA, Cuba, Russia, Africa, India and the UK. Rather than using professional models in her editorials, Hawkins tends to take pictures of either friends or strangers she spots on the street (who often end up becoming friends), seeking out men and women with a particular appearance or style. Though influenced by the work of cult American photographer Diane Arbus, she does not seek to position her subjects, no matter how extreme, as outsiders or 'other', but gives them the space and time to revel in their personal style and celebrate their individuality. American photographer Tina Barney's elaborate domestic tableaux could also be cited as a more recent influence, while French photographer Lise Sarfati's suburban female subjects provide another, more contemporary point of reference.

Fashion is a carefully considered part of Hawkins's images. She photographs her subjects in their own clothes but also collaborates with stylists. While her sitters may not always choose their outfits, she makes sure that they are never uncomfortable. Once again, we see here an emphasis on the potential for self-expression and play through dress up.

An important aspect of Hawkins's practice is her own participation as subject. She has posed alongside male models in a 2008 Versace campaign for *i-D* and appeared as an iconic country music singer in a 2011 story for *PonyStep*. For this second project, 'Dolly Parton is my Religion', she photographed herself in various situations dressed as Parton with the singer's trademark big, blond hair (which is actually very similar to her own). One self-portrait taken in the mirror in which she holds the camera to her eye reminds us of the artifice of the images. This is Hawkins as both photographer and fan playing the role of the country music singer and perhaps questioning how Dolly sees herself.

Hawkins's images have been widely published and exhibited. The influential magazine editor and stylist Katie Grand is a huge supporter of her work, which featured regularly in *Pop* and continues to appear in Grand's latest project, the Condé Nast biannual *Love*. Hawkins has also produced extended editorial for the relatively new *PonyStep* magazine. Her commercial clients include Agent Provocateur, Häagen-Dazs, Topman, Diesel, Tommy Hilfiger and Cos.

---

82 'Christina Madrid Green' from 'Miss East Anglia', *Citizen K*, 2007 — **84** 'Self-Portrait as Page Three Girl', *i-D*, 2007
85 'Holly Madison with Lady Macbeth, Playboy Mansion' from 'Alice's American Safari', *Pop*, 2008 — **86 above** 'Dominga and Isabel, Cuba' from 'Another Country', *Love*, 2012
86 below 'Jeffery Wilson' from 'Nairobi', *Love*, 2011 — **87** 'Dolly Parton is my Religion', *PonyStep*, 2011 — **88** 'Ckapura Hulle Banepoebha' from 'From Russia with Love', *Pop*, 2007
89 'Jackie Gordon and Aaron Smith with Peanut the Chihuahua, Las Vegas' from 'Carlo's World', *PonyStep*, 2013

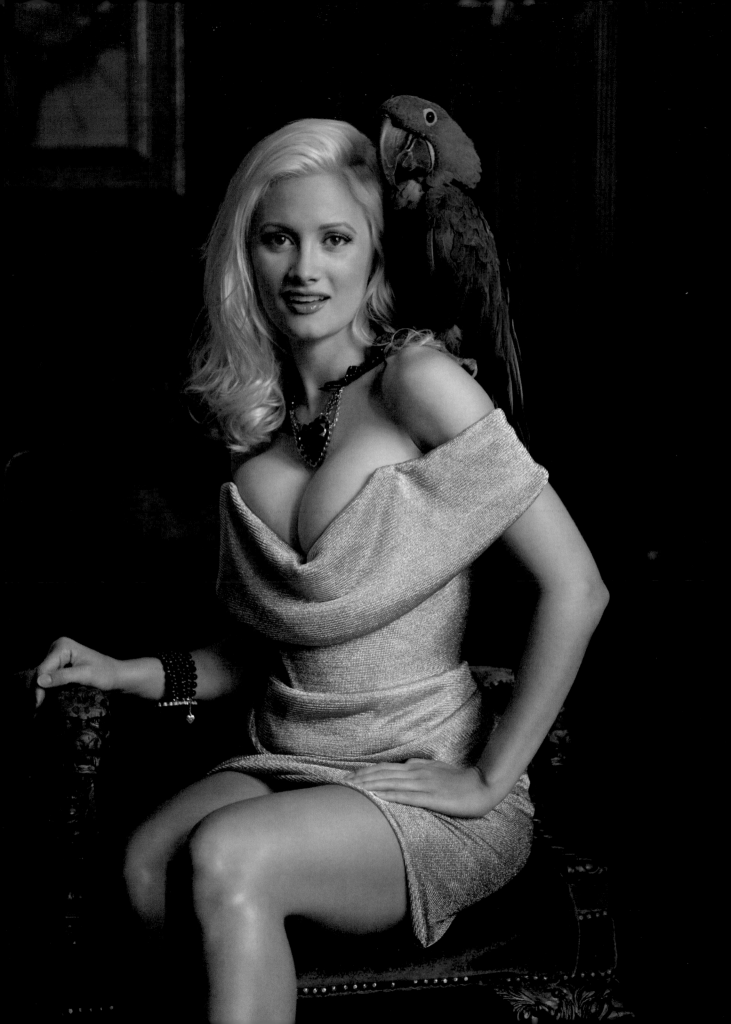

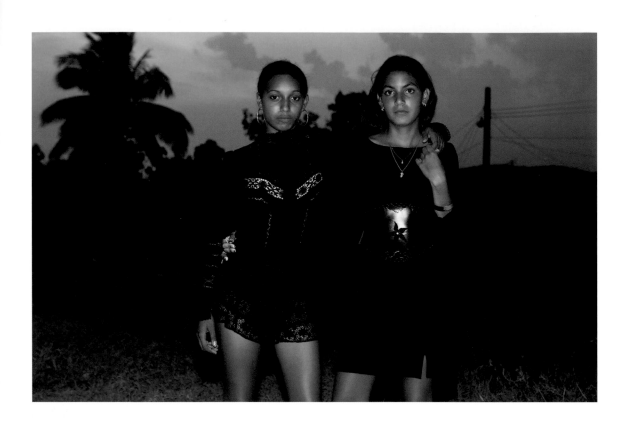

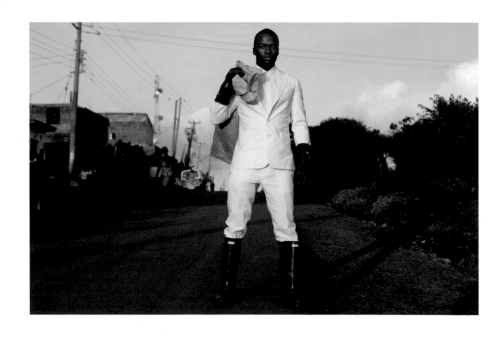

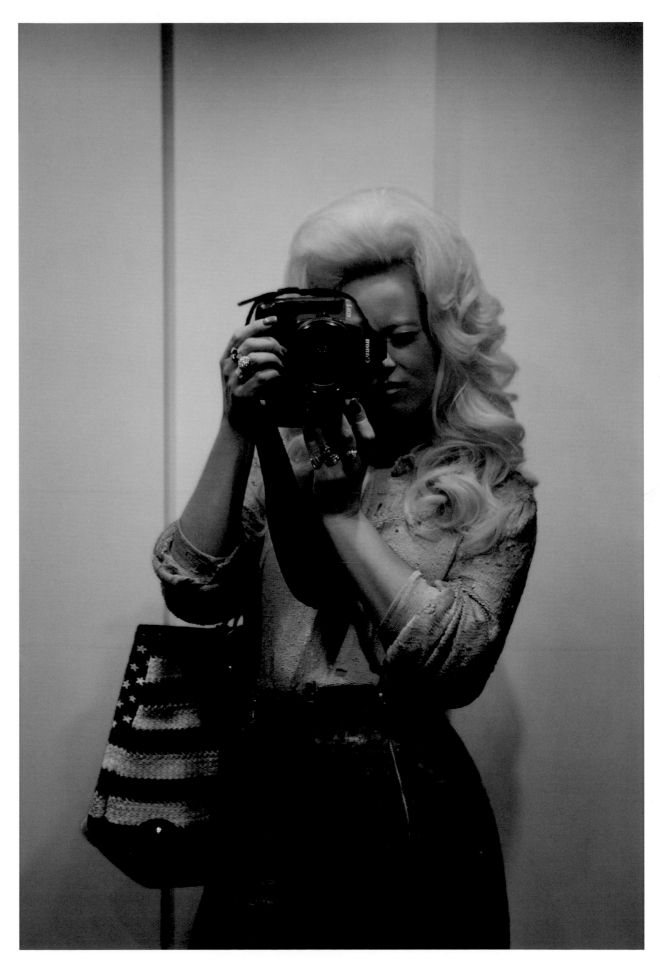

Alice Hawkins

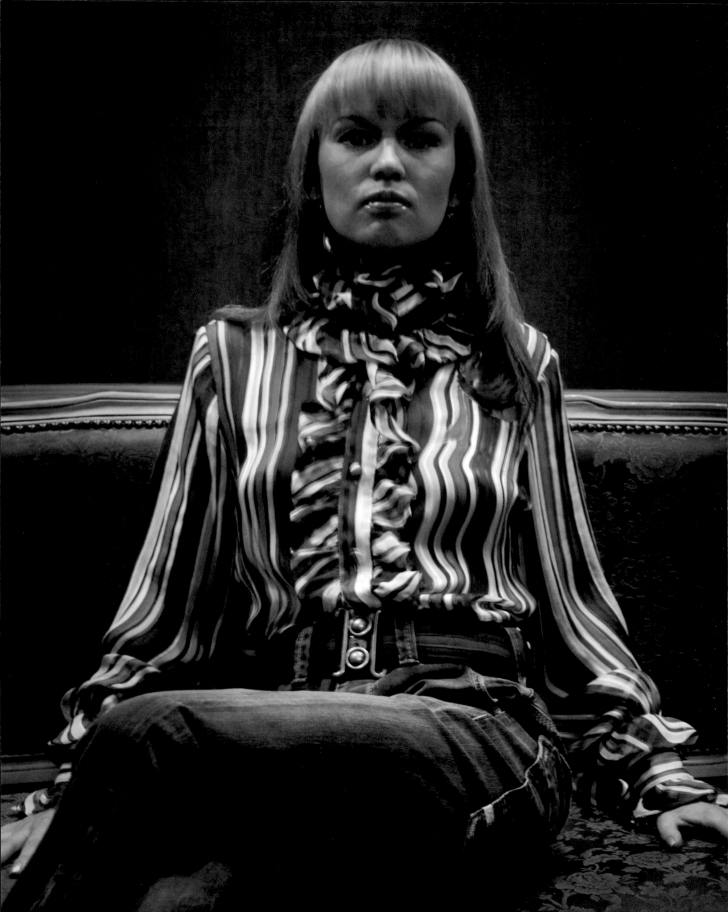

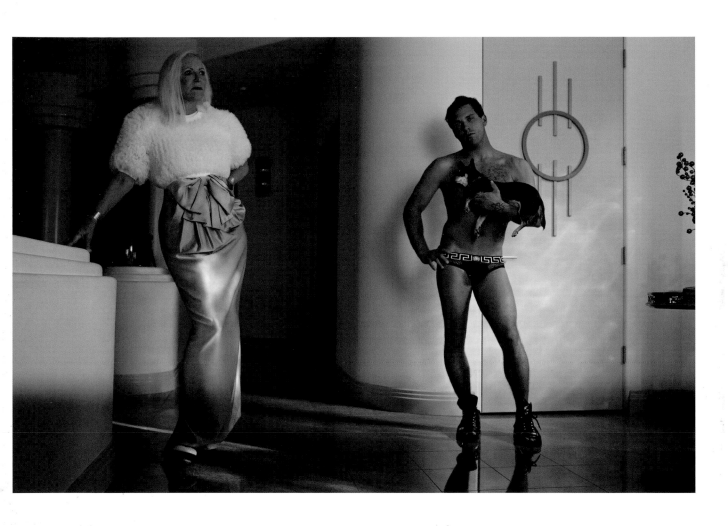

Alice Hawkins

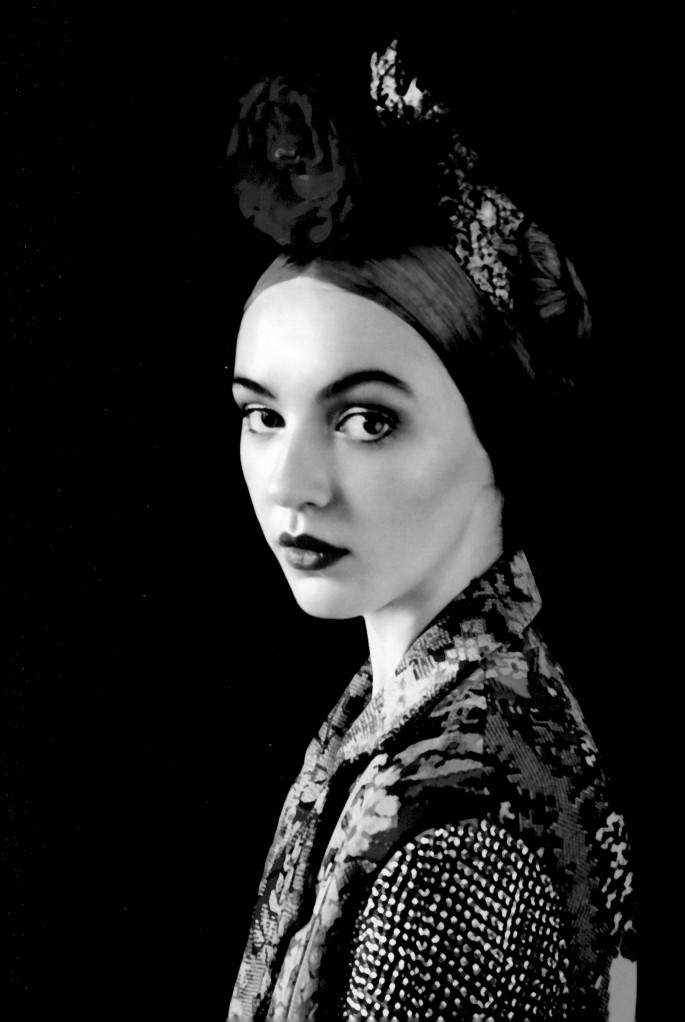

Erik Madigan Heck's multi-faceted creative process involves painted sets, in-camera effects and digital post-production.

Erik Madigan Heck

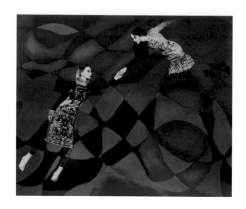

Erik Madigan Heck (b. 1983) is an American photographer who works between London, Paris and New York, where he is primarily based. Born in Excelsior, Minnesota, he was given a 35 mm Canon camera by his mother when he was 14 and began taking photographs soon after. He holds a BA in political science from Salve Regina University in Rhode Island and an MFA in photography and film-related studies from Parsons School of Design in New York.

In 2012, Heck was the youngest photographer ever to be commissioned for the prestigious Neiman Marcus 'Art of Fashion' campaign. The following year, he was the recipient of the 29th Infinity Award for Applied/Fashion/Advertising. He regularly appears on 'Ones to Watch' lists – he was featured in *Forbes*'s '30 Under 30: Art & Design', for example, as well as in *The New York Times*. Despite these numerous accolades, Heck's greatest achievement is the staunch determination with which he follows his unique creative vision and his joyful propensity to take risks in order to make a different statement with each new project. This is something of an anomaly in high fashion, where commissioners often

require photographers to produce images within a narrow style or range for which they subsequently become well known. Heck's photographs and short films dare to differ from what he has made previously, as well as from the work of his contemporaries. They are conceptualized as responses to a designer or collection rather than a single garment.

Heck's diversity can be seen in an ongoing collaboration with the London-based, Greek designer Mary Katrantzou. Covering all five seasons since autumn/winter 2011, the photographs are published in *Nomenus Quarterly*, the limited-edition magazine with a free online edition founded and edited by Heck himself. The first project with Katrantzou, 'Surreal Planes', was both hyperreal and unreal, a play between flat surfaces and sculptural forms. In one image, the brilliantly saturated hues of the two-dimensional patterned background echo the designer's vivid, three-dimensional printed fabrics. Heck has described his interest in achieving painterly effects in his photographs. By carefully orchestrating pose and framing, and by altering the negative or print with analogue and digital techniques, he creates compositions that often cleverly reference historical portrait paintings.

Heck's creative process is multi-faceted, beginning with a simple concept and later involving painted sets, in-camera and on-set effects, darkroom manipulations and digital post-production. In a photograph from the second project with Katrantzou, 'The Surrealist Ideal', two female models are transformed into paper dolls against what looks like a hand-painted blue patterned background in a dreamlike composition reminiscent of a Marc Chagall painting. For the fourth project, 'Murals', Heck makes use of strong silhouettes and in one image creates a backdrop of Egyptian hieroglyphics that once again references Katrantzou's prints. He strips away all colour in the fifth project, 'Cathedrals'. Here, the models are more ethereal, fading away into darkness in a reversal of some of the earlier projects, where the figures appeared to sit on top of the bright patterns.

Heck has collaborated with many other significant designers, including Ann Demeulemeester, Haider Ackermann and Dries Van Noten. Like many new generation photographers, he is not restricted by traditional perceptions of what fashion images should look like, but instead strives to make expressive and beautiful pictures.

---

90 'Florals' from 'Nature vs Nurture' for Mary Katrantzou, S/S 2012 — 92 'Blue Flying Study' from 'The Surrealist Ideal' for Mary Katrantzou, A/W 2012
93 'The Art of Fashion' for Neiman Marcus, 2012 — 94 above & below 'Interior Study' and 'Portrait' from 'Surreal Planes' for Mary Katrantzou, A/W 2011
95 'Collage' from 'Murals' for Mary Katrantzou, S/S 2013 — 96–97 'The Art of Fashion' for Neiman Marcus, 2012

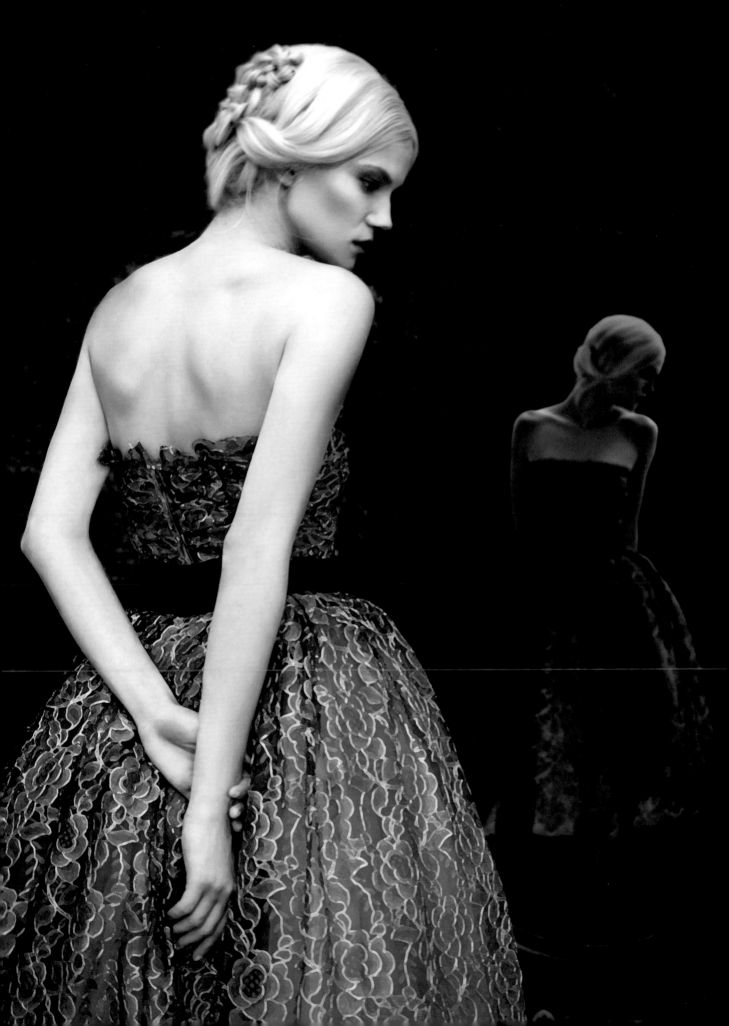

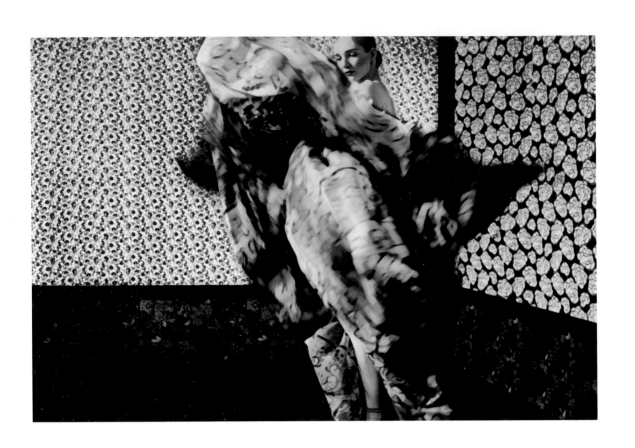

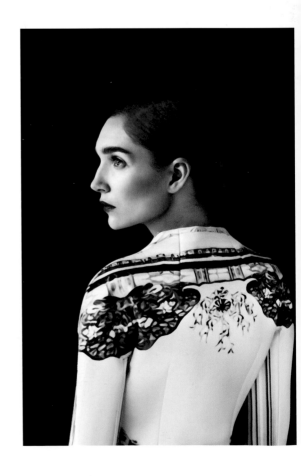

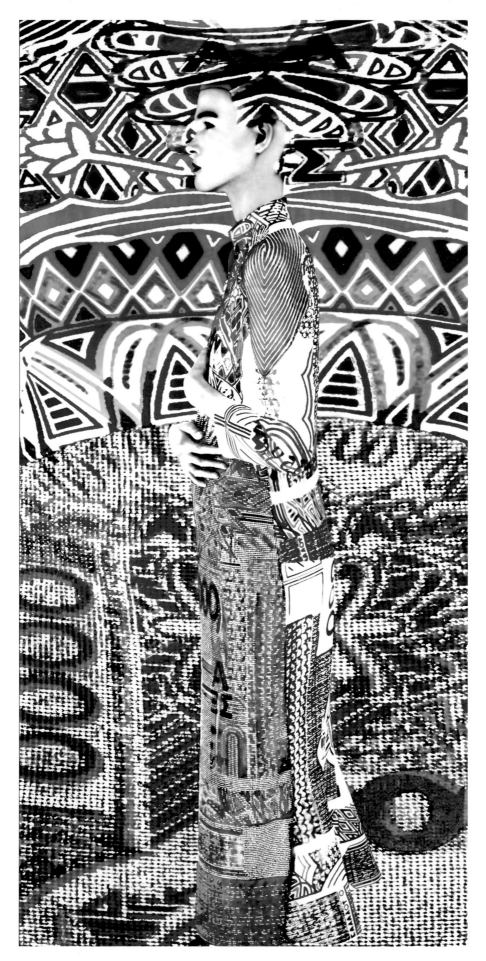

Erik Madigan Heck

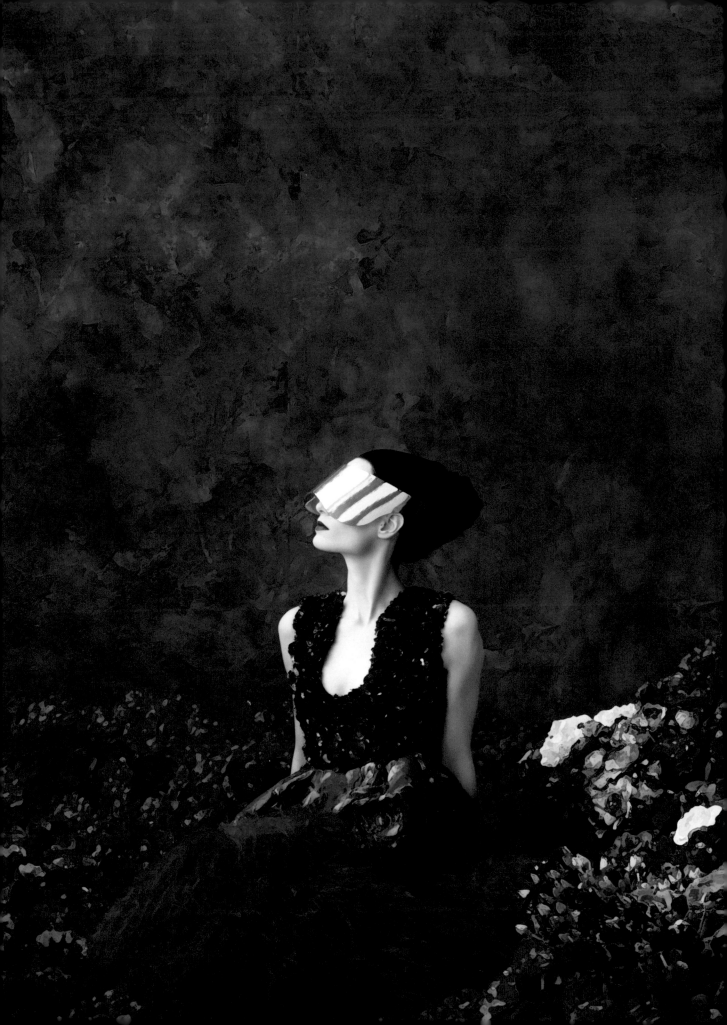

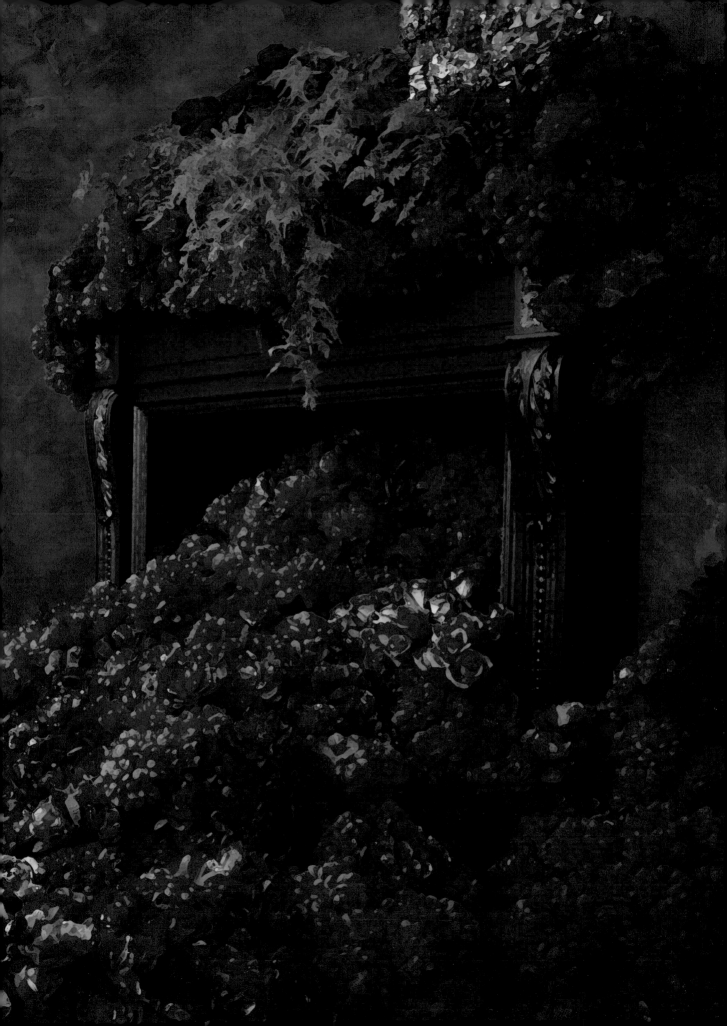

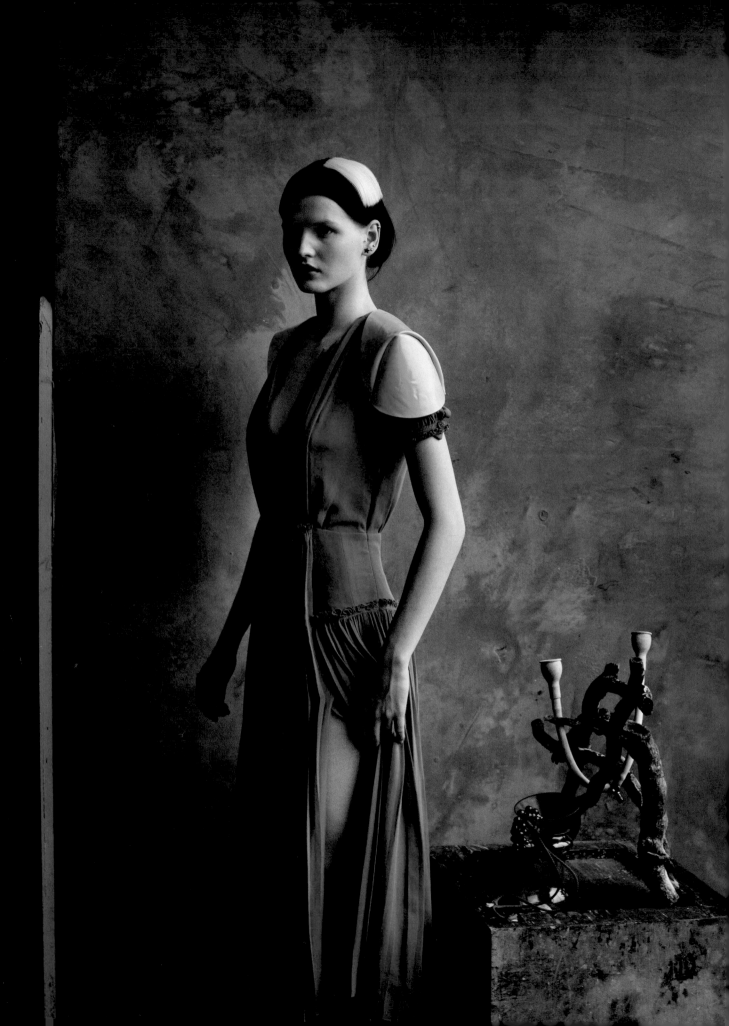

Julia Hetta's images are filled with a sense of gravitas and weight; they are still rather than fleeting.

Julia Hetta

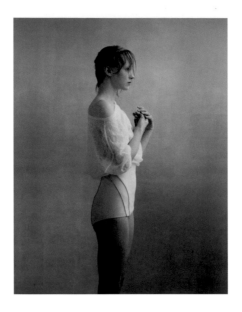

Julia Hetta (b. 1972) is a Swedish photographer based in Stockholm who also works extensively between London and Paris. She has been interested in photography since her childhood: her father, a doctor, set up a darkroom in the family home. During her 20s, Hetta worked for five years as a researcher at a photography agency. While there, she was immersed in the medium, examining many thousands of prints, and she considers the experience to be crucial to her particular understanding of image-making. She subsequently embarked on a formal training, completing a three-year degree in photography at the Gerrit Rietveld Academie in Amsterdam in 2004.

After graduating Hetta did not assist but began working with her brother, the stylist Hannes Hetta, who at the time was a fashion editor at *Vogue Hommes International*. He remains her most important collaborator. Together, they have made what she describes as 'our universe, our own language', working in the studio to produce editorial and brand advertising for clients such as *Dazed & Confused*, Chinese *Vogue*, *The New York Times*, *Le Monde* and Hermés. 'Jungfrukällan' for *Acne Paper* in 2011 was an important breakthrough for the sibling duo and featured many of the stylistic elements that set Hetta's photographs apart from her contemporaries: rich colour hues; a dramatic use of light and shadows, with models often emerging from or receding into dark backgrounds; and an overwhelming impression of composure and containment – what Hetta has termed 'silence'. Thomas Persson, editor-in-chief and creative director of *Acne Paper*, has been a significant commissioner, and the large-scale A3 format and heavy matt paper of his publication have proved to be an inspired platform for Hetta's work.

Hetta's images are filled with a sense of gravitas and weight; they are still rather than fleeting. Indeed, her studio process is slow and considered with low light and long exposures. Even when working digitally, she does not shoot quickly or profusely but approaches each click of the shutter as though it were about to create an important picture. This unhurried deliberation is manifest in the stylized poses of her models, in the intricate arrangements of limbs, and purposeful gestures and expressions. Other stories with stylists Cathy Edwards (for *AnOther*) and Mattias Karlsson (for *Acne Paper*) have featured more of a narrative, yet Hetta disrupts these surreal, dreamlike fantasies with flashes of colour – brilliant pinks, blues and yellows in backgrounds, or in models' garments or makeup – that jolt us back to the here and now.

Although it is not difficult to see why Hetta's photographs are often likened to historical paintings, this is also a superficial comparison. It is certainly not the main intention of her approach, which is shaped equally by the history of photography and her own imagination and desire to tell stories. Her clever and sometimes joyfully inexplicable still-life compositions act as abstract counterpoints to the figure studies, functioning in the same way as the vivid colour in her portrait work. With these still lifes, we are once again reminded that we are looking at a world of Hetta's own making, rather than a pastiche of a moment in the past.

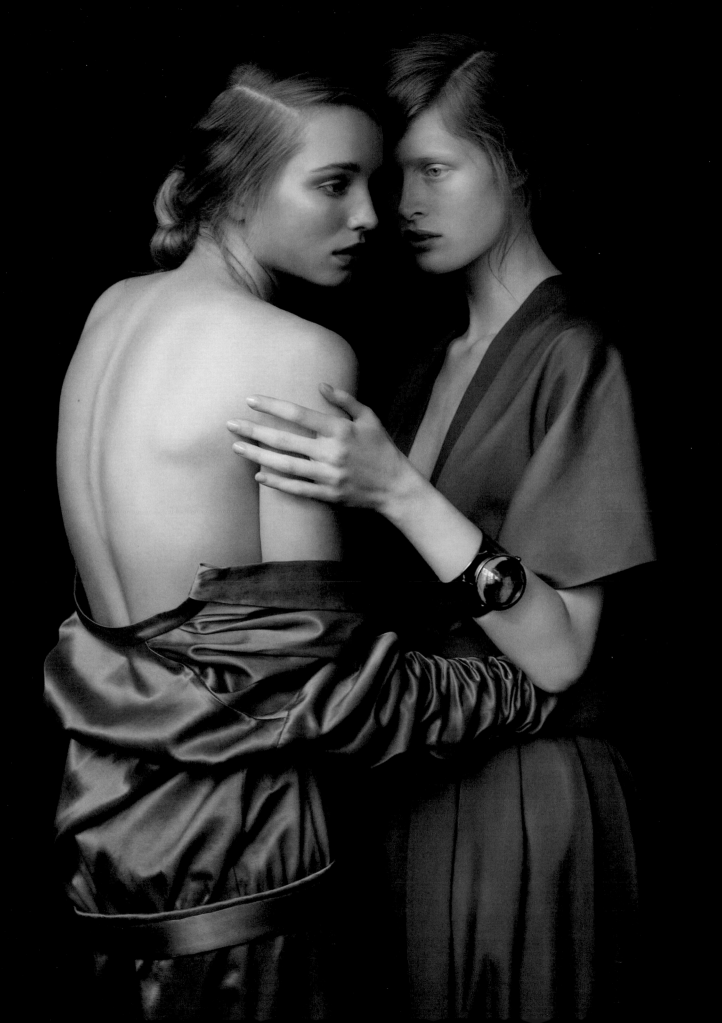

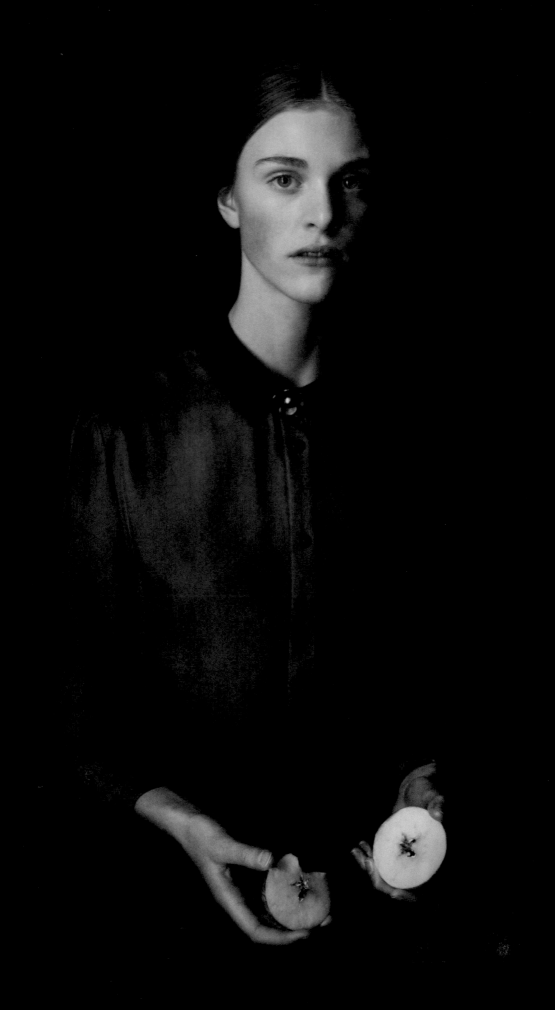

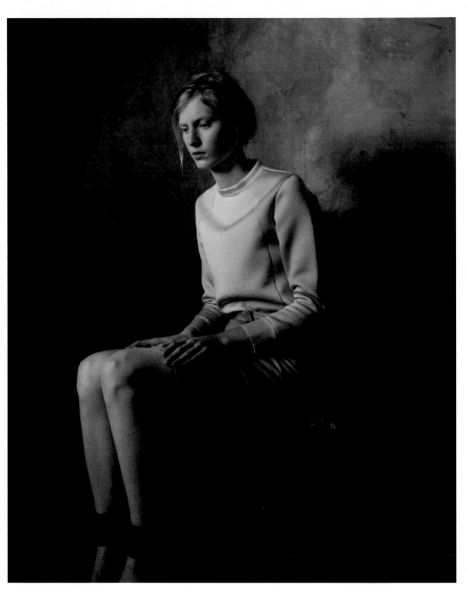

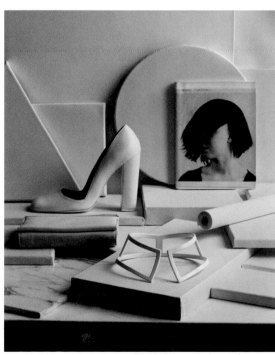

Julia Hetta

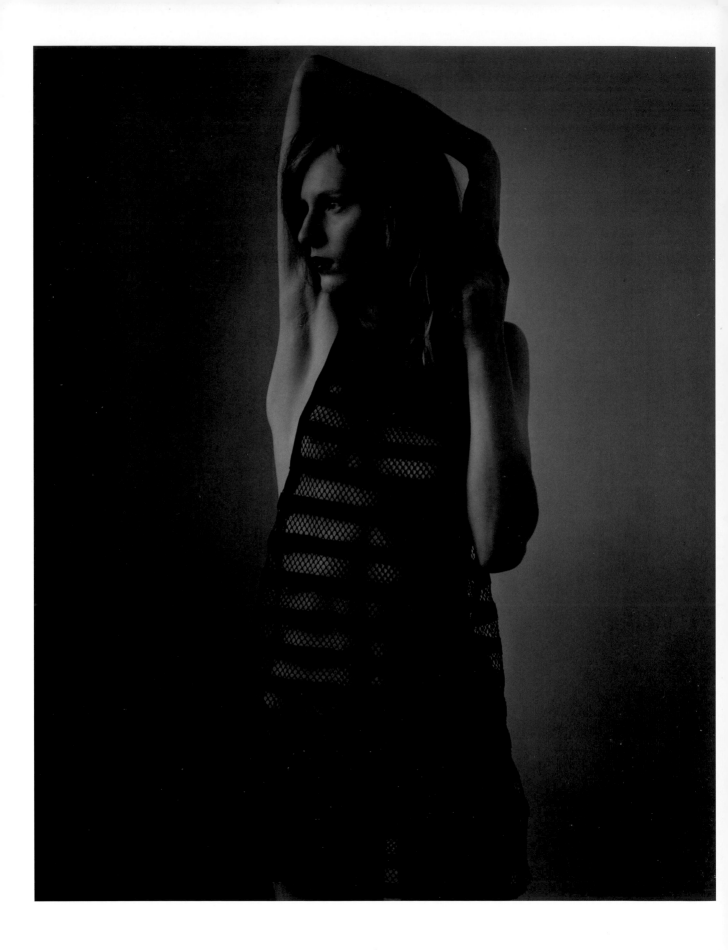

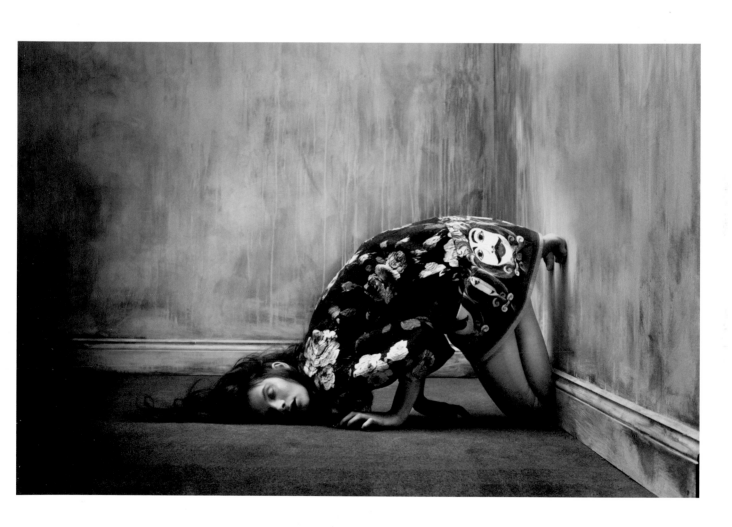

Julia Hetta

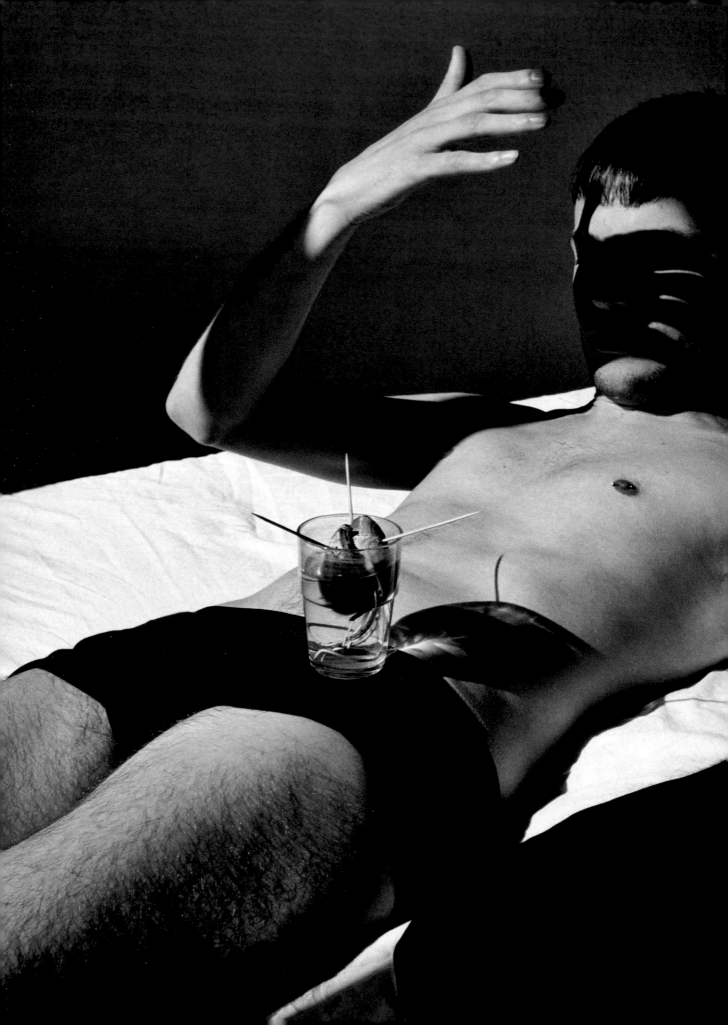

Samuel Hodge's practice mixes diaristic documentation with idyllic, hazy fantasy.

Samuel Hodge

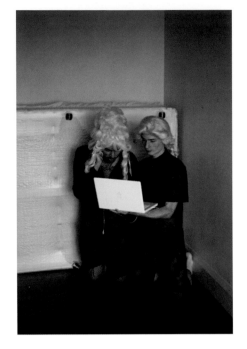

Australian photographer Samuel Hodge's (b. 1978) exclusively analogue practice exists somewhere between diaristic documentation and idyllic, hazy fantasy. He grew up in Glen Innes, a town of about five thousand people in rural New South Wales, before relocating to Sydney in 1997. Three years later, he started taking photographs, often referencing gay pornography but translating it into art photography – see, for example, his zine *Truth/Beauty/Cock* from 2005.

By the late 2000s Hodge had moved into fashion, and since travelling to Europe in 2010 he has been working between cities, building up an international presence. His photographs have appeared in numerous magazines (from *Yen*, *Russh*, *Dazed & Confused* and *Oyster* in Australia to *I Love You*, *Weekday*, *Die Zeit* and *Butt* in Europe), as well as in books (*Pretty Telling I Suppose* was published by Rainoff in 2009) and self-published dossiers (*Sometimes I Just Need Quiet*, 2008). In addition, Hodge has exhibited his work in art galleries and at one-off events in Sydney, Paris, New Orleans and Berlin, where he is now based. He has also collaborated with such leading fashion brands as the eclectic Australian design duo Romance Was Born.

The world Hodge creates is at once highly personal and poignantly universal.

His images frequently feature long shadows and models with obfuscated visages in ambiguous poses or halfway gestures. He often photographs friends or lovers, lending a very personal kind of intimacy to his images, especially those in which he captures his models looking directly at the camera. This technique of simultaneously revealing and obscuring his subjects invites the external viewer to contemplate figures that are both uncannily familiar and totally elusive. As such, Hodge's work seems to be about the personal and universal experience of fleetingness and the unstoppable passage of time. This sense of nostalgia for a moment always-past is not only tangible in the images themselves, fashion or otherwise; it is also evident in Hodge's approach to photography in general.

Hodge never studied photography and he admits to not being interested in the technical side of the medium – in cameras, or printing and developing processes. He has never worked digitally and always uses the same equipment, preferring to take pictures with old SLRs from the 1960s and '70s. His unskilled approach stems from his disregard for new technology, as well as from his preoccupation with and prioritization of the moment of shooting itself. Whether sitters are long-time friends or models he has just met, there is always an intuitive nonchalance to the way Hodge works with his camera to capture people. He rejects the need to plan his images and does not construct scenarios or set up artificial lights and other equipment and props in advance. Instead, he always uses natural light, looking for locations that allow for the ultra-dark silhouettes, muted tones and unexpected pools of light that are central to his aesthetic. The shoots usually take place indoors in domestic spaces – in his own home or at friends' apartments – both out of expediency and for familiarity with the light. This explains the proliferation of photographs documenting his family home and its surroundings.

Lately, however, Hodge has started working more in outdoors locations. To his surprise, he has discovered that he is very capable of shooting in bright sunlight as well as indoors. Recent projects, such as an unpublished story made with Australian Aboriginal model Samantha Harris in 2012, suggest that his eye for the moment translates well into non-domestic spaces, perhaps indicating a new direction in his work.

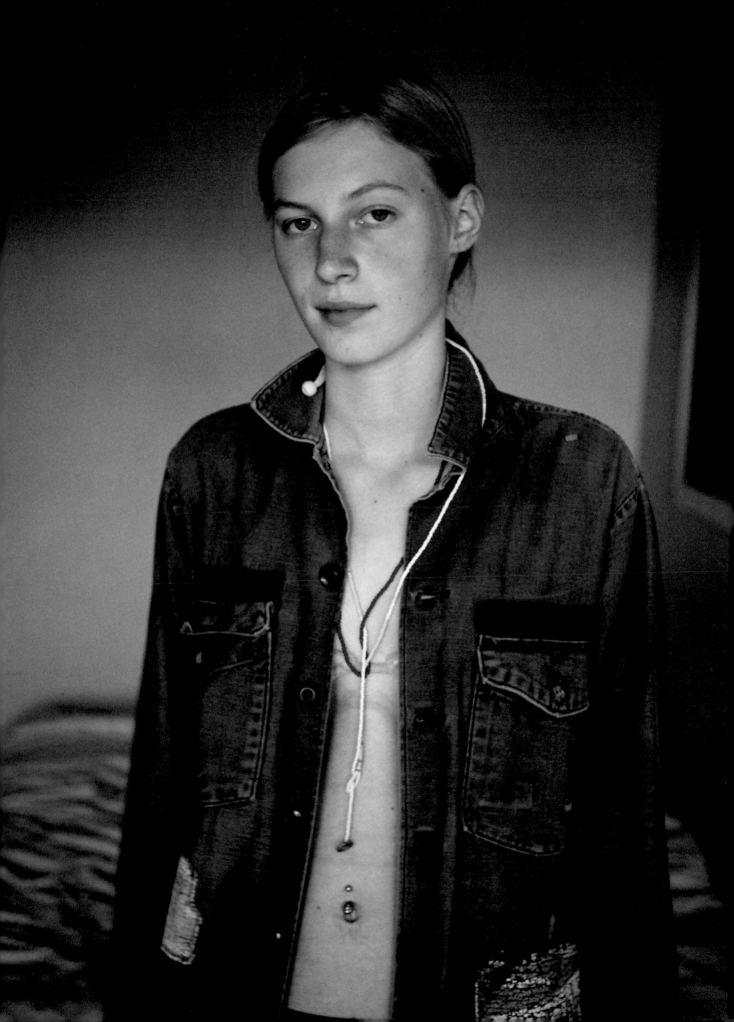

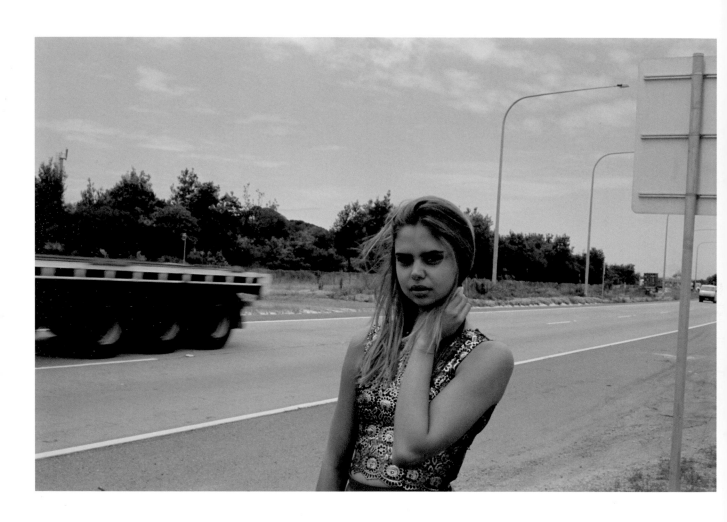

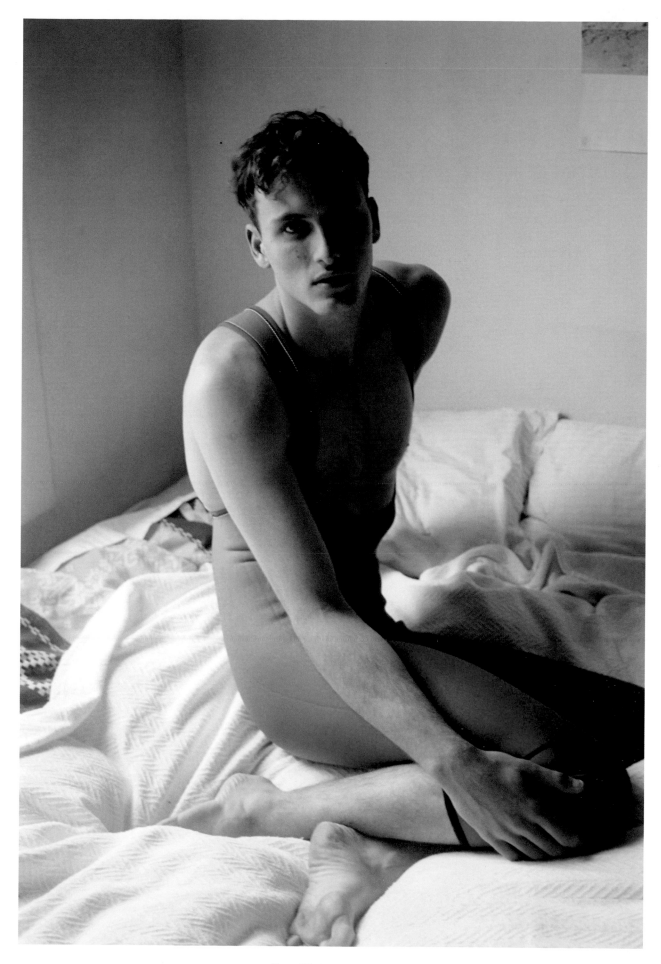

Samuel Hodge

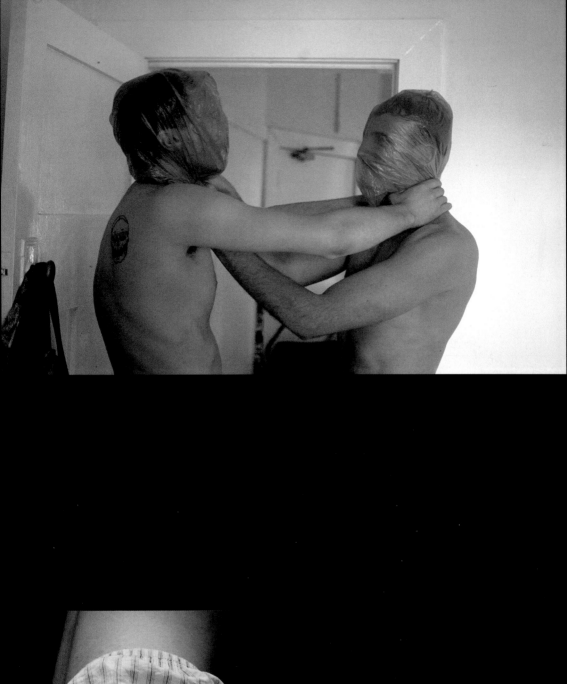

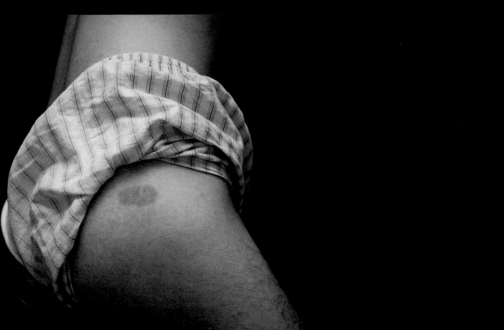

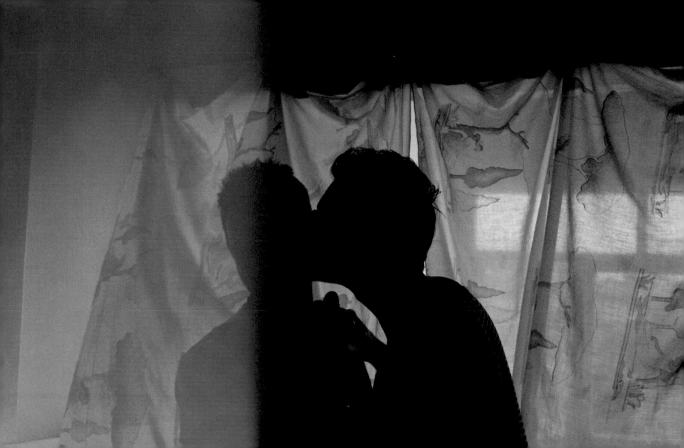

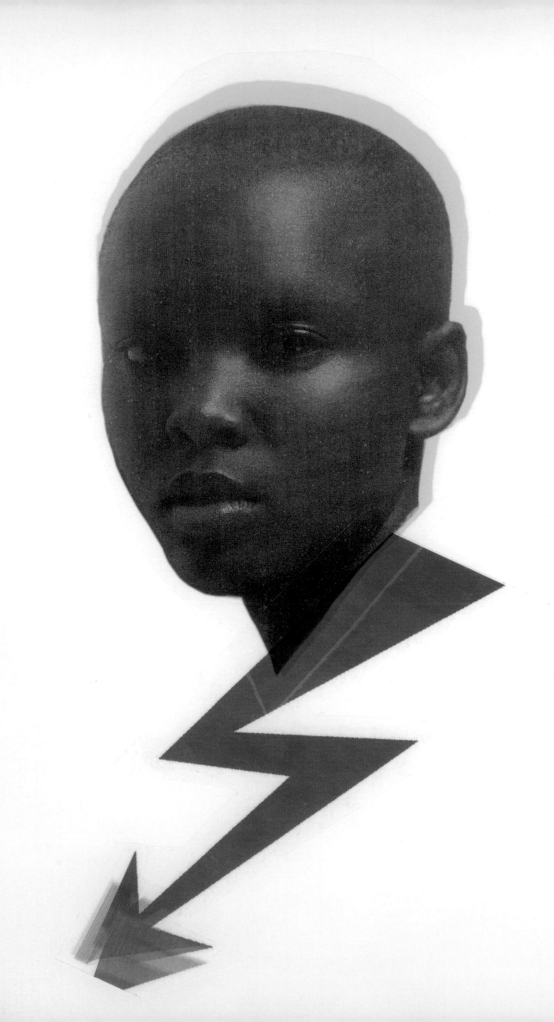

Axel Hoedt's aesthetic derives from his persistent exploration of analogue processes.

Axel Hoedt

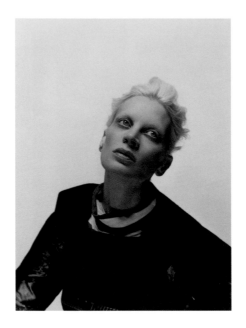

Axel Hoedt (b. 1966) is a German photographer who is based in London. He studied photography under Karl Martin Holzhäuser and Gottfried Jäger at the University of Applied Sciences in Bielefeld, Germany, where he was particularly influenced by Jäger's theories on abstract composition. Since arriving in London in 1998 Hoedt has worked extensively in fashion, cultivating an unusually sustained independent vision. His practice is considered and intelligent, and his straightforward, often black-and-white images significantly extend the trajectory of contemporary studio fashion photography. Contrary to expectation, Hoedt's particular aesthetic derives from a persistent exploration of analogue processes and equipment, rather than an exploitation of digital technology.

Hoedt works in the studio with a large-format film camera and also makes considerable use of Polaroid. He obtains additional effects and manipulations both in-camera and during the developing and printing processes. As a result, his pictures can be atmospheric, even romantic in tone, yet he often disrupts the fragile, dreamlike perfection of traditional fashion imagery by embracing and including mistakes, and by employing techniques such as double exposure and composite negatives. He receives many commissions from avant-garde designers whose creations require his alternative aesthetic and unorthodox construction of beauty.

Rather than aspiring to create seamless, abstract spaces, Hoedt encourages the viewer to consider the limits of the studio. In one image from 'Into the Light', an Alexander McQueen feature shot for *i-D* magazine in 2011, the brilliantly cast Tanzanian model Flaviana Matata is posed stopped short by the studio wall with her back to us. Hoedt reminds us that his studio is a constructed, physical working space by leaving black electrical tape markings on the floor that become graphic compositional lines in his images. In the same story, Matata faces Hoedt in a cropped, three-quarter-length portrait. Here, the softer horizontal lines across the photograph look like shadows cast on set, but are in fact a second layer of visual effect created in the darkroom by applying a separate exposure and negative to the print.

Another project with the experimental designer J. J. Hudson, who transforms found garments into masks and headpieces, started out as a feature for *Pop* magazine under the editorship of Katie Grand. Hoedt approaches his fashion commissions as a photographer first, so what would normally have resulted in one or two pictures taken over the course of an afternoon morphed into a larger project that saw him photograph Hudson and his assistant wearing the masks at his own Hackney studio and the designer's Brighton base. The images relate to another series begun around the same time on the Fastnacht festival, an annual, pre-Lenten carnival in southern Germany involving costumes and masks. Though the two series are unconnected, the Fastnacht images are also studio portraits, made using the same methods and equipment, in which masquerade and performance complicate the conventional studio documentation or straight, descriptive presentation of costume and dress.

114 Flaviana Matata, 2011 — **116** Kristen McMenamy, *Archivist*, 2013 — **117 & 118 above** Anouk Hagemeijer, *Zoo International*, 2009
118 below Abbey Lee Kershaw, *i-D*, 2011 — **119** 'Into the Light', *i-D*, 2011 — **120–121** 'NOKI', 2007

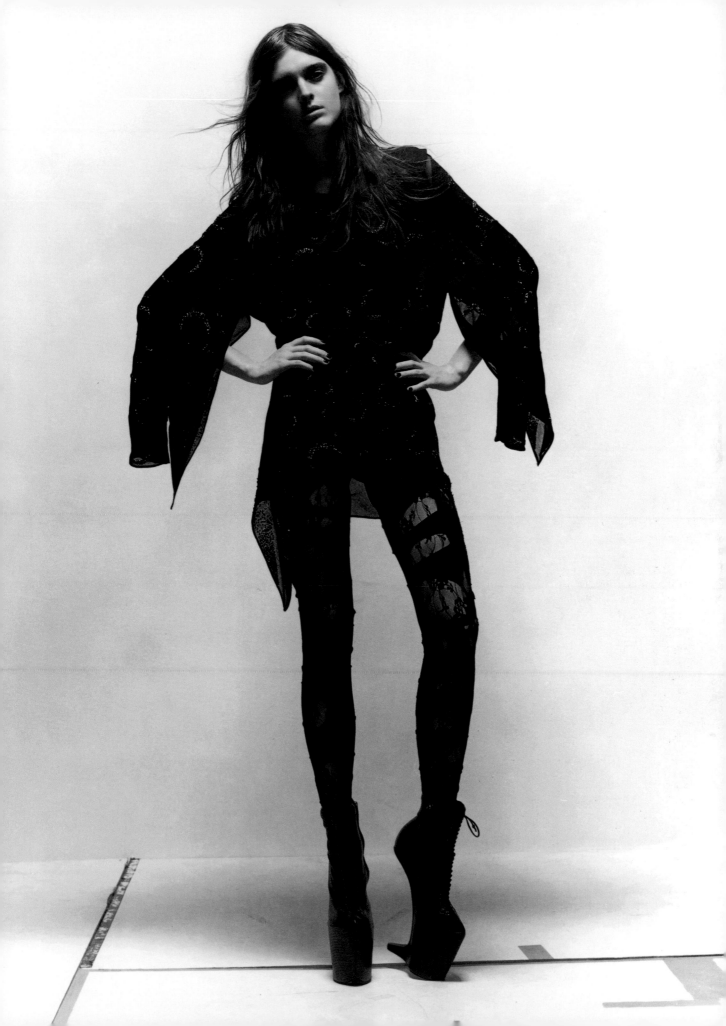

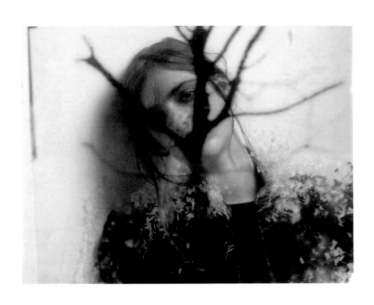

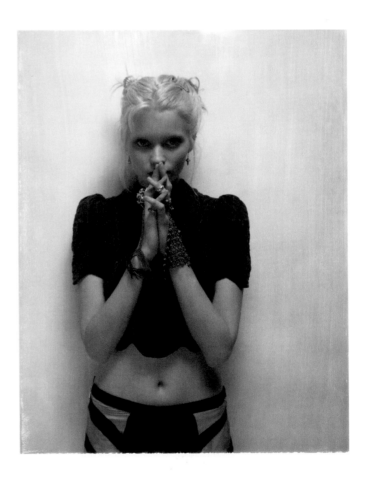

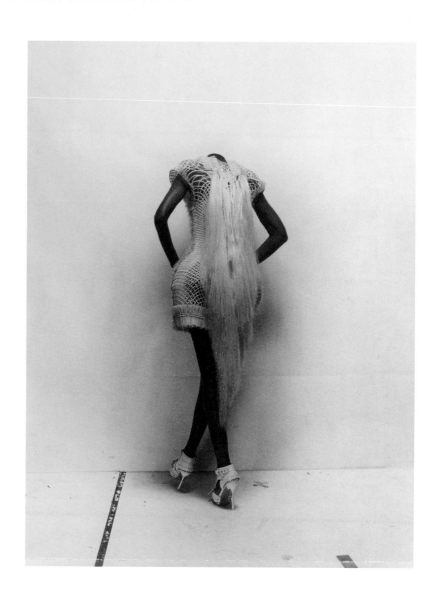

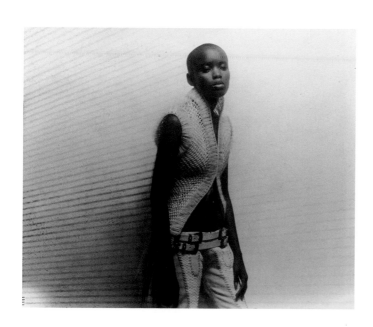

Axel Hoedt

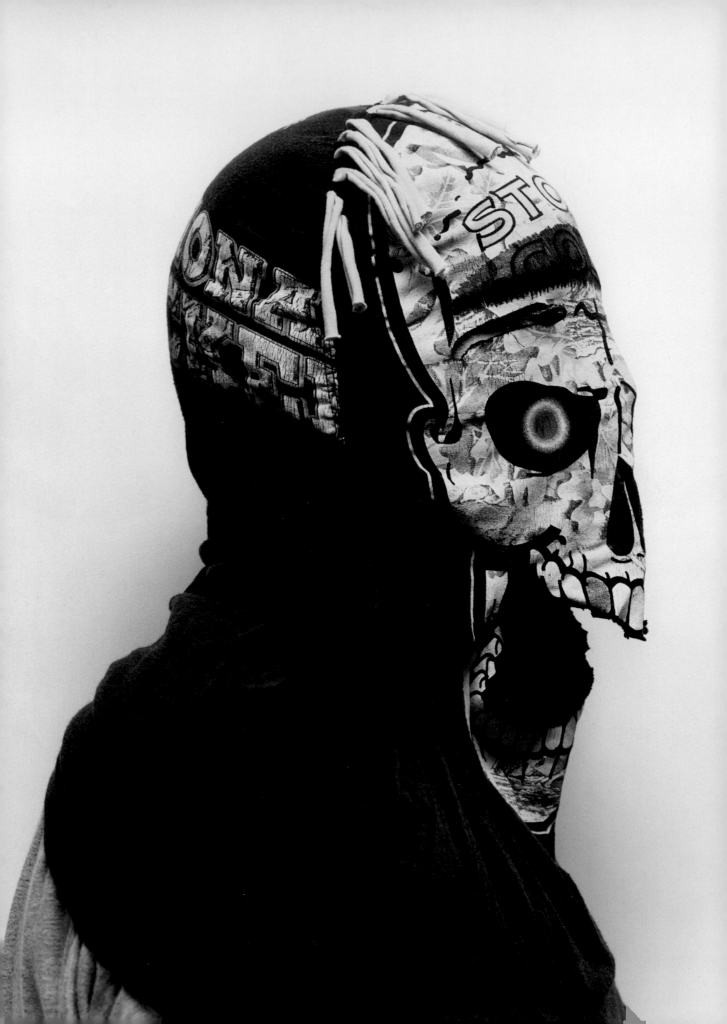

Laetitia Hotte's detached compositions are often free from context or background narrative.

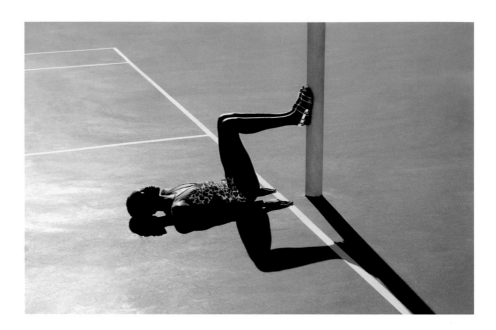

French photographer Laetitia Hotte (b. 1982) is one of the newest talents in this book. In 2004, after completing a degree in photography and graphic design, she moved to Paris to continue her studies with a focus on photography at the Ecole Nationale des Arts Décoratifs. Hotte first worked in fashion not as a photographer's assistant but as an art director and designer at various French magazines, including *Jalouse* and Olivier Zahm's progressive *Purple*, both important platforms for emerging art directors and photographers. She continued to take photographs after finishing her studies, however, and her first fashion images were published in *Jalouse* in 2009 and *L'Officiel* in 2011.

Hotte is predominantly a studio photographer, working with 35 mm film and digital cameras. Her photographs have a compelling sense of disconnect: unlike many fashion images, besides the basic elements within the photo frame, her compositions are often totally free from any form of context or background narrative, lending them both a strangeness and a formalism. This impression of cool detachment distinguishes Hotte's work from that of her contemporaries and is undoubtedly grounds for further experimentation.

Hotte often plans her shoots on mood boards in advance. Reflections, shadows and other compositional effects are obtained in-camera, often with the help of mirrors and other props, but she also uses post-production from time to time. Movement and shape are an important part of Hotte's work and she is especially influenced by dance, in particular the work of visionary American choreographer William Forsythe. She cites American photographer William Eggleston as another formative influence; this is most evident in her use of strong colours.

In 2013, Hotte received her most important commission to date from the Japanese label Kenzo. She has a particular fascination for contortionists and used them in the shoot to model a range of forest and orchid-print garments against a simple, bright-blue background. The resulting poses cleverly confound our sense of the beginning and end of the garments and the bodies they adorn. Although these poses were necessarily orchestrated in order to create certain shapes, the final photographs are no less expressive and energized than more spontaneous or movement-based fashion images. Indeed, while Hotte's deliberateness – her emphasis on stiff and formal poses – might have been unfashionable in editorials of recent years, it is now an aesthetic that sets her work apart as distinctive and bold.

———

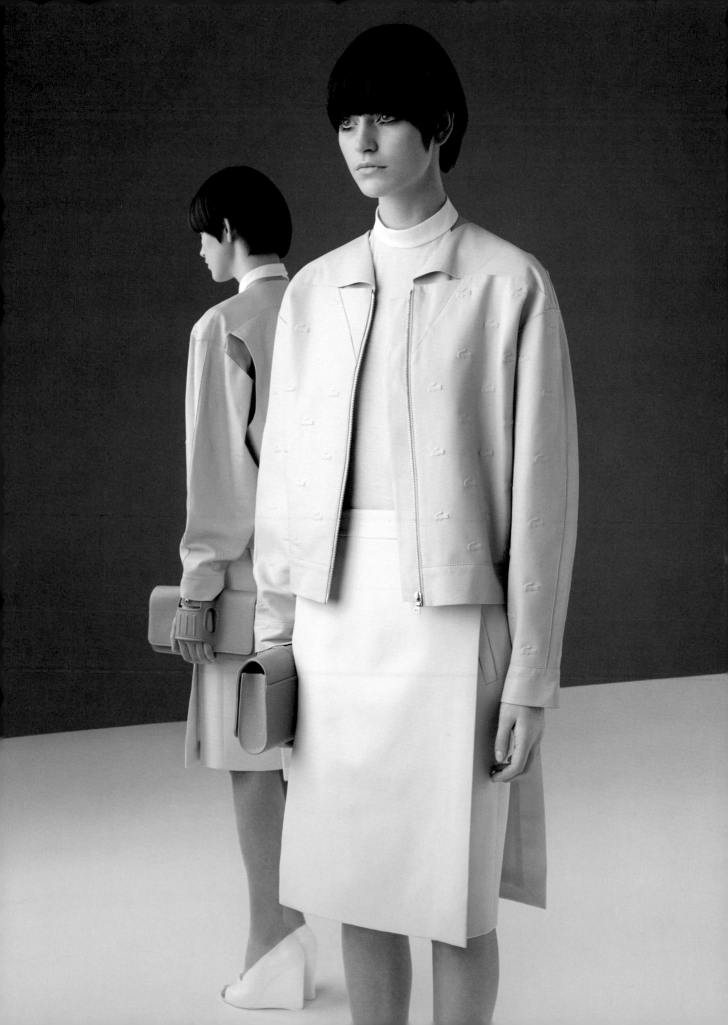

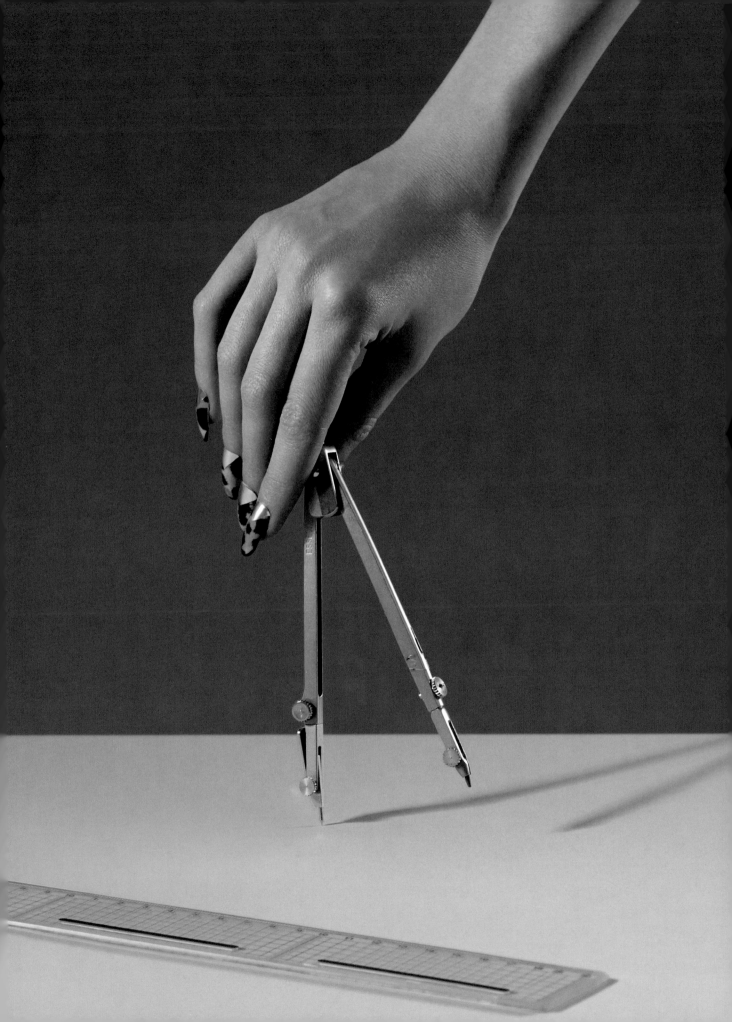

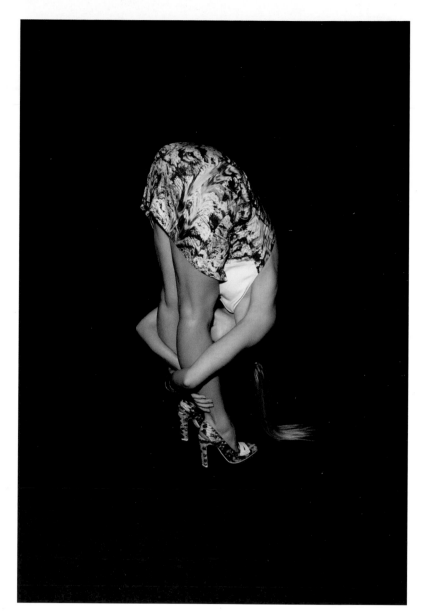

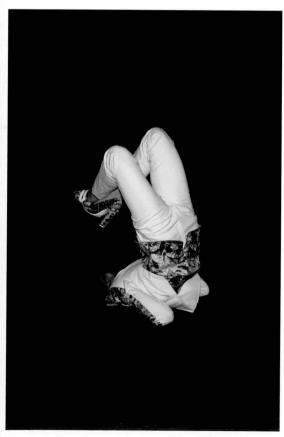

Laetitia Hotte

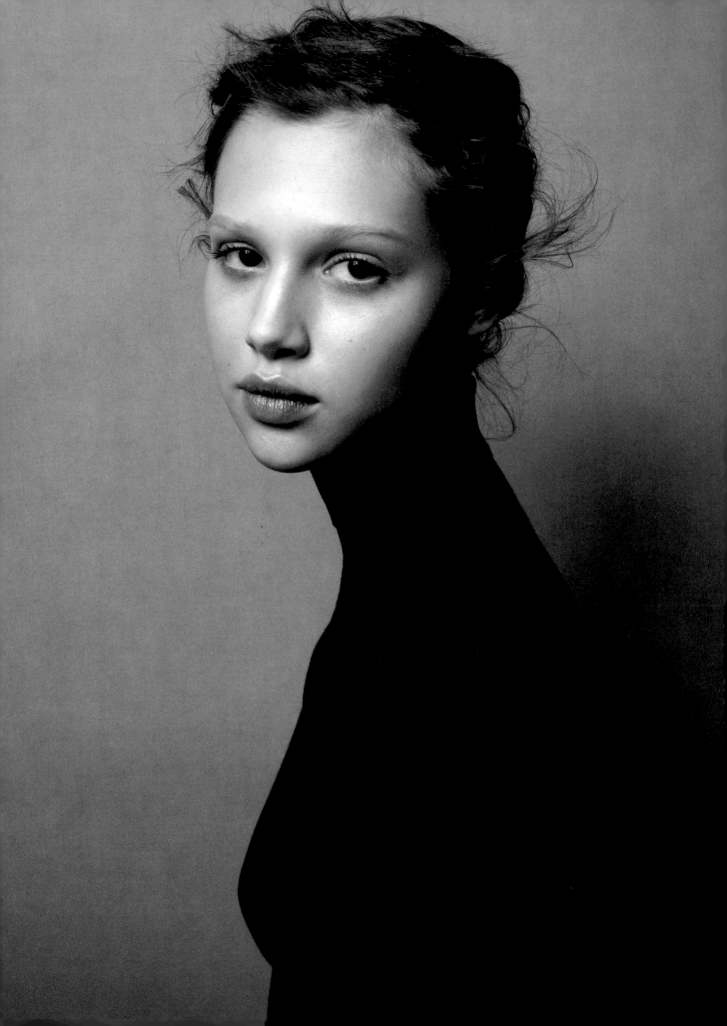

Daniel Jackson is one of the most outstanding, exciting and in-demand figures in fashion photography.

Daniel Jackson

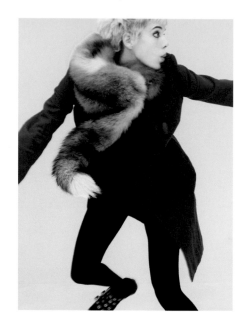

Daniel Jackson (b. 1976) is a British photographer based in New York. Although he trained as a sculptor – he holds a BA in fine art from the Chelsea College of Arts in London – Jackson has been interested in photography since the age of 11, when he was given his first camera. Influenced by style magazines such as *The Face* and *i-D*, which were significant cultural touchstones for many young artists in the 1990s, he began to work increasingly with photography, particularly portraiture. In 1999 he moved to New York, where he spent eighteen months working first as a studio assistant and subsequently as a photographer's assistant. He returned to London in 2001 and the following year took a job with David Sims, one of the most important fashion photographers of the last thirty years.

Jackson began working independently in 2005 and almost immediately was commissioned to produce editorial features for *Dazed & Confused*, *i-D* and *Purple*. Fashion magazines often run stories by emerging photographers who then may or may not receive more work, depending on their ability to create innovative features that express the concept of a collection while adhering to the style and position of the publication. Since his very first commissions, Jackson has continued to produce exemplary campaigns and editorials for various international publications. He has become one of the most outstanding, exciting and in-demand figures in contemporary fashion photography.

Jackson's photographs are frequently, but not exclusively, shot in the studio. Dynamic movement is a brilliant stylistic feature of his work, a transformative visual tool he consistently employs to create dramatic shapes that bring the garments to life. In an early picture from 2006, for example, the British model Agyness Deyn – whose classic red coat and fur scarf are updated by Samira Nasr's Brit Punk styling, with spiked hair, black leggings and studded ankle boots – could be making a dash for a bus on a central London street. A 2007 location shoot for *Self Service* includes an image of the Italian model Mariacarla Boscono balancing on one leg with her arms pushed out to one side, enhancing the top half of the frame and the colourful styling by Marie Chaix. In a photograph from a 2012 feature for *AnOther* styled by Katie Shillingford, the Norwegian model Erjona Ala strides forwards, highlighting the bold contrast of colour and texture – from shoes to tights to leggings – and accentuating the overall look via the swing of the outer cape.

A compelling aspect of Jackson's work is his ability to convey successfully the different personalities and attitudes of his models. As a result, what are ostensibly fashion pictures also function as portraits or character studies. 'Spring Forward', for example, which was published in British *Vogue* in 2012, was a collection story on a diverse group of fashion designers. Jackson was nevertheless able to create a visual link between the designers by shooting the clothes in unadorned studio settings. It was as though the garments were the models' own and he was exploring his subjects' individual styles.

In 'Persona', styled by Mattias Karlsson for *Acne Paper* in 2011, models became method actors posing for intense portraits. A similar sense of theatricality was evident in previous collaborations with Karlsson for *Acne Paper*: in the debauched 'It's My Party' from 2010, for instance, which was about youthful decadence and lost innocence; and in the stunning nude study 'Tradition' from 2008, a more painterly love story. In both editorials, the development of the narrative relied on the creation of strong characters across the image sequence.

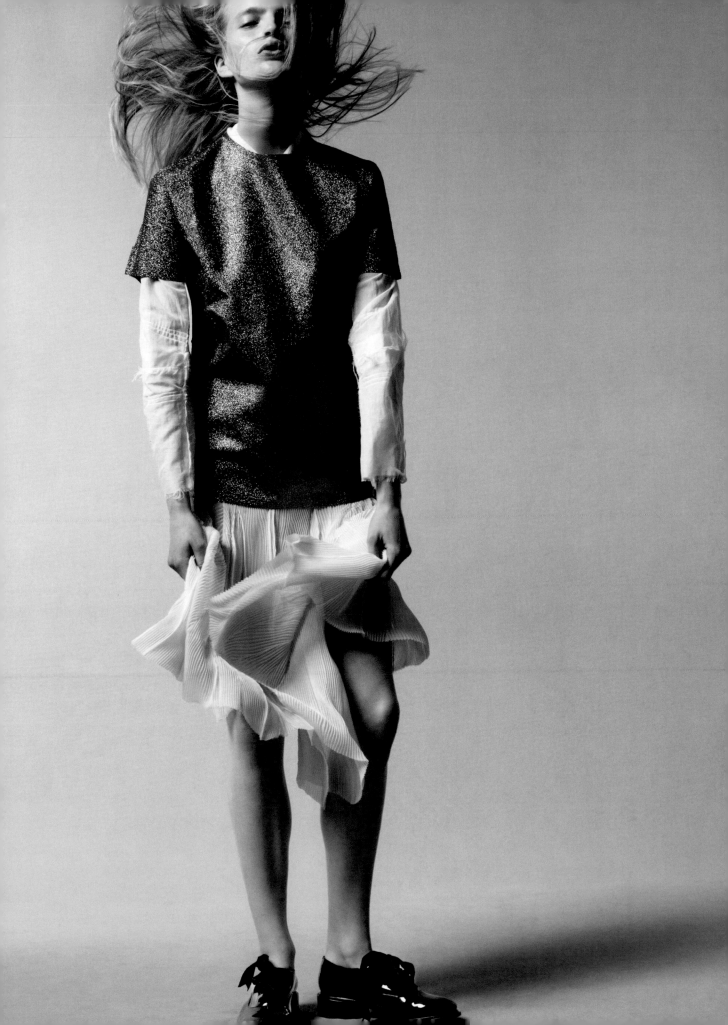

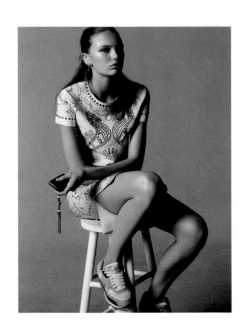

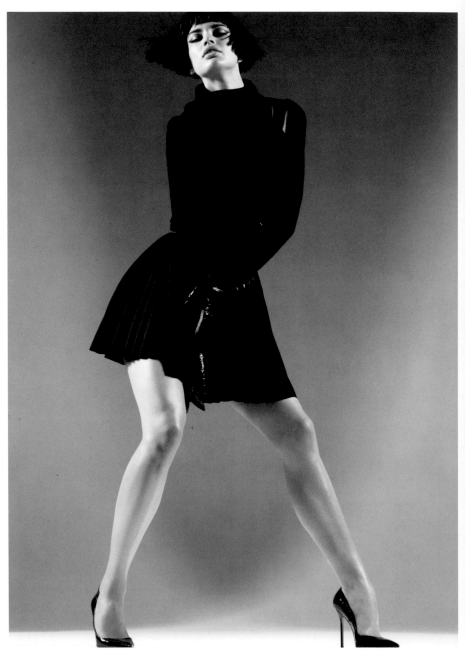

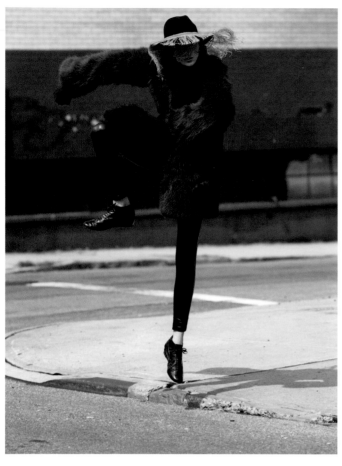

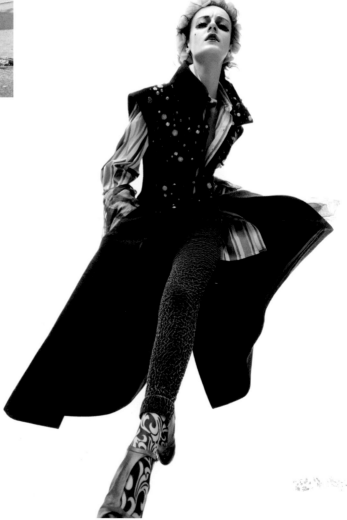

Daniel Jackson

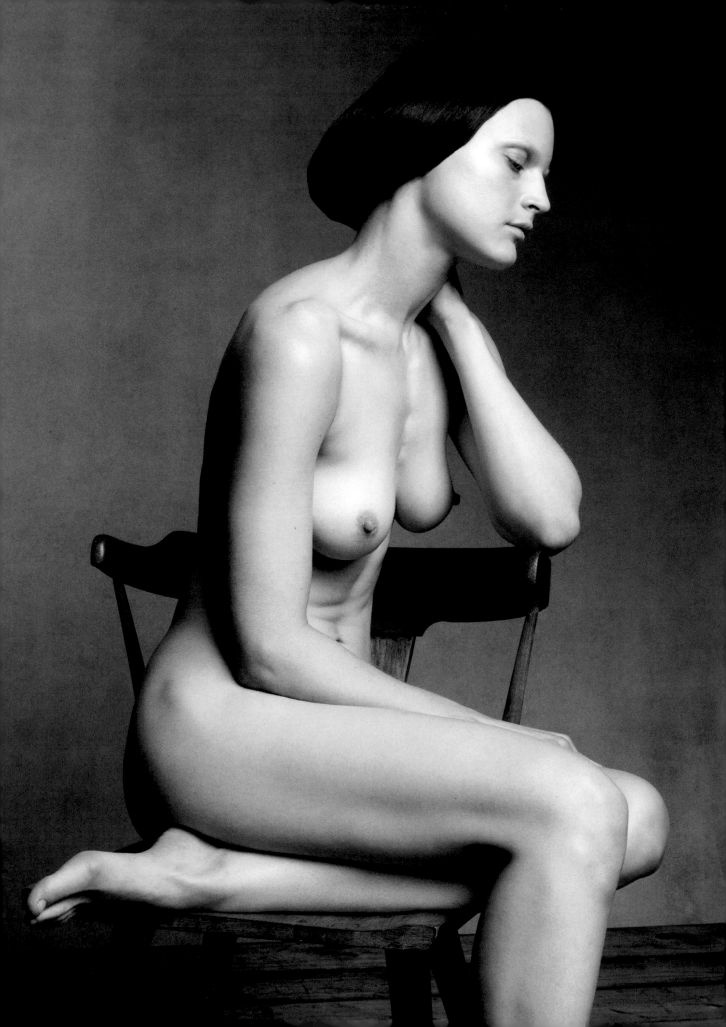

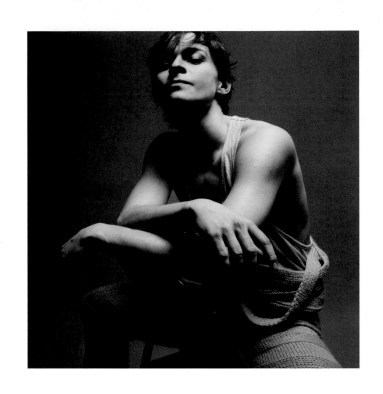

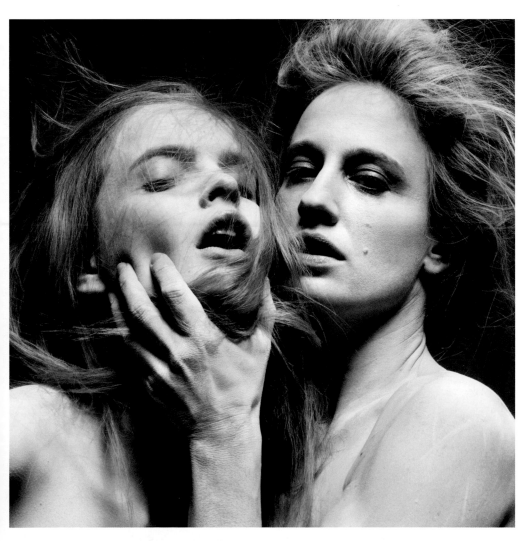

Daniel Jackson

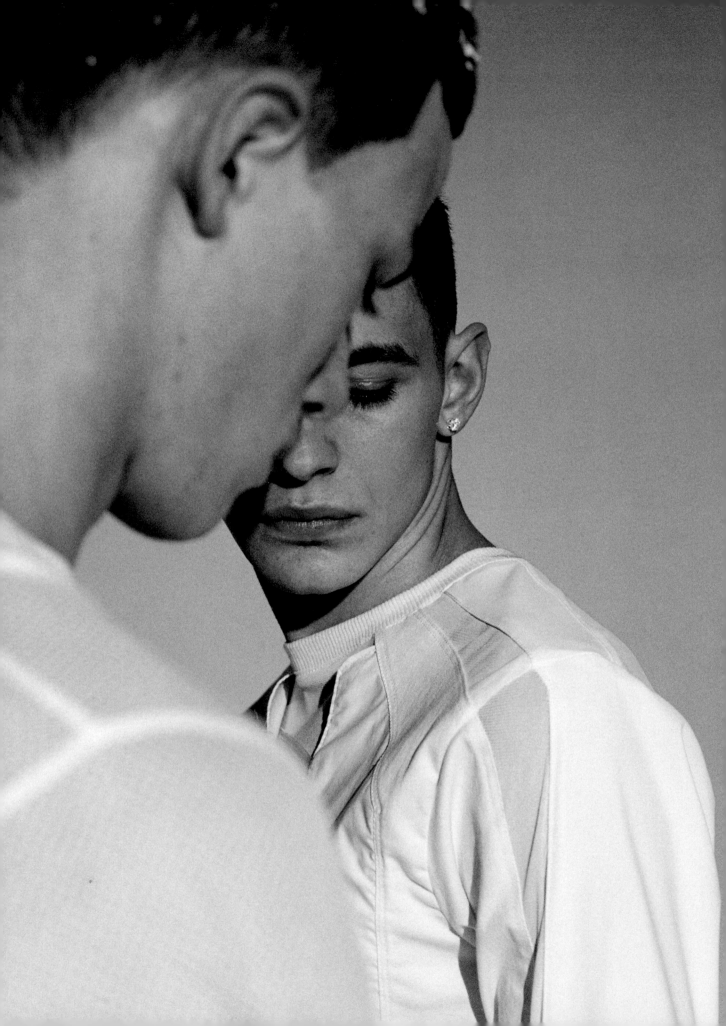

Bruna Kazinoti's work has a strong graphic quality and sometimes a gritty urban realism.

Bruna Kazinoti

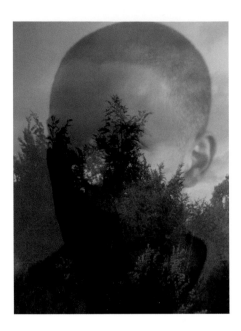

Bruna Kazinoti (b. 1983) is a Croatian photographer. She is based in Split but also travels between London, New York and Paris. She studied photography at the Royal Academy of Fine Arts in Antwerp, where she worked closely with the university's fashion department, which is renowned for its progressive design and the calibre and later success of its students. Her end-of-degree project was a portrait study of her then boyfriend, and much of her subsequent editorial work has focused on men's fashion and the male subject.

Men's fashion photography, traditionally less prevalent in the history of the genre, had a resurgence in the late 1990s and early 2000s. Many new men's style magazines – *Arena Homme +*, *GQ Style*, *Man About Town*, *Fantastic Man* – were established, reflecting the conceptual interests of a group of photographers and stylists who were redefining the representation of masculinity and male sexuality in fashion editorial. A student during this period of exceptional creativity, Kazinoti was inspired by some of the leading figures in men's fashion,

including photographers David Sims, Alasdair McLellan, Benjamin Alexander Huseby and Willy Vanderperre (who also studied at the Royal Academy of Fine Arts in Antwerp), and stylists Simon Foxton and Olivier Rizzo. As a female photographer making a significant contribution to men's fashion, Kazinoti is a rarity in her field.

Kazinoti's first break came in 2008 with an editorial styled by Katie Shillingford for *Dazed & Confused*. Like almost all of her work the story was shot with a Nikon camera on 35 mm film, although in this case she created an arresting tactility by combining two images – photographs of landscapes and sculpture with portraits and fashion stills – during post-production. Since then, her work has been published in *Pop*, *Tank*, *Arena Homme +*, *L'Officiel Hommes*, *Oyster*, *Hero*, *Rebel* and *Qvest*.

Like several of the photographers in this book, Kazinoti's approach tends towards the personal and the intimate. She is confident working with artificial lighting in the studio – as in her 2011 story 'Sports +' for *Arena Homme +*, for example – but she

also frequently shoots outdoors with natural light. While the overall direction of her editorials is planned in advance, her photographs are often defined by the way the models move on set, which may be a more unexpected outcome of the shoot. This spontaneity should not imply a softness or sense of nostalgia, however; Kazinoti's work has a strong graphic quality and sometimes a gritty urban realism.

Kazinoti is another emerging photographer with little interest in pursuing the dominant aesthetic of the fairytale fashion narrative (which involves working with top models in the studio and impossibly perfect retouching during post-production). Shape and pose are relaxed in her images though not always naturalistic, particularly when choreographed for compositional purposes. Kazinoti frequently photographs models from behind, suggesting, perhaps, a rejection of some of the traditional modes of fashion image-making: the face is almost as important in fashion photography as it is in portraiture.

136 'Sports +', *Arena Homme +*, 2011 — 138 'Antwerpen Malik', 2008 — 139 'Salt Water', *Oyster*, 2012
140 above 'Sins and Sensibility', *Tank*, 2012 — 140 below 'To the Power', *Rebel*, 2011
141 *Pop*, 2010

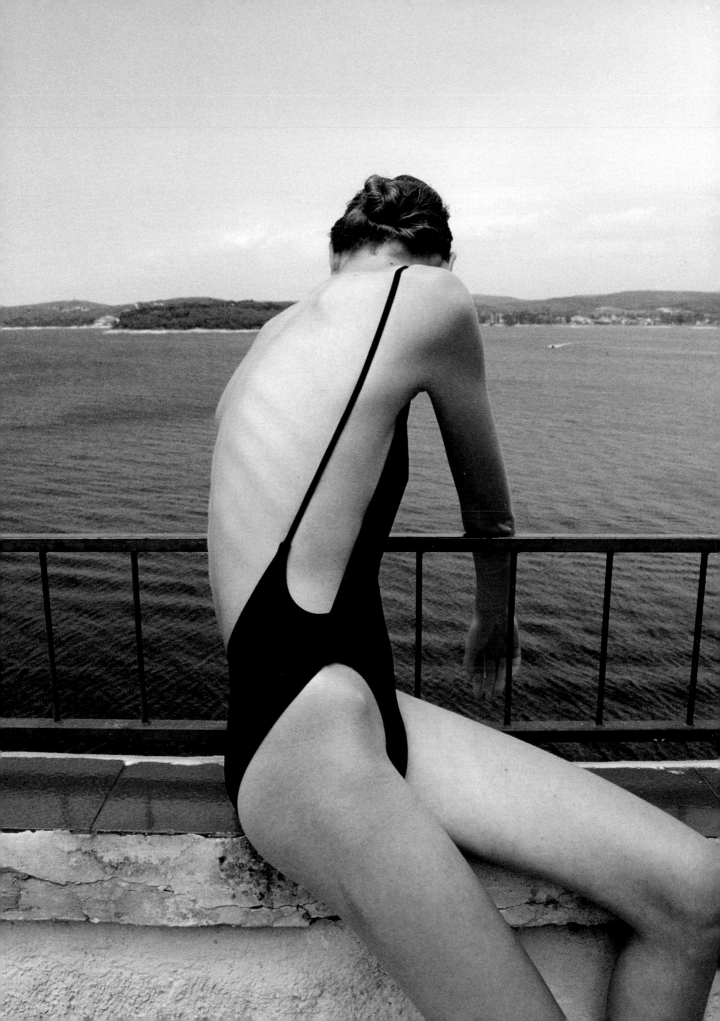

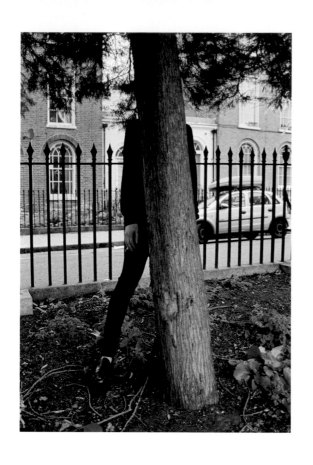

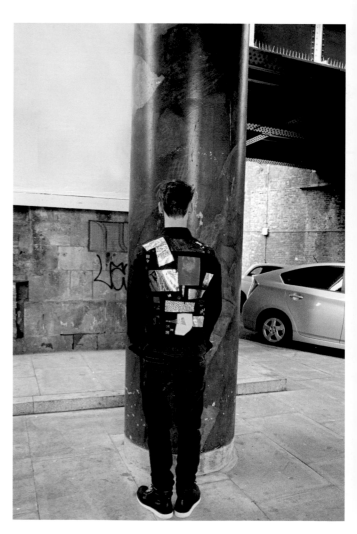

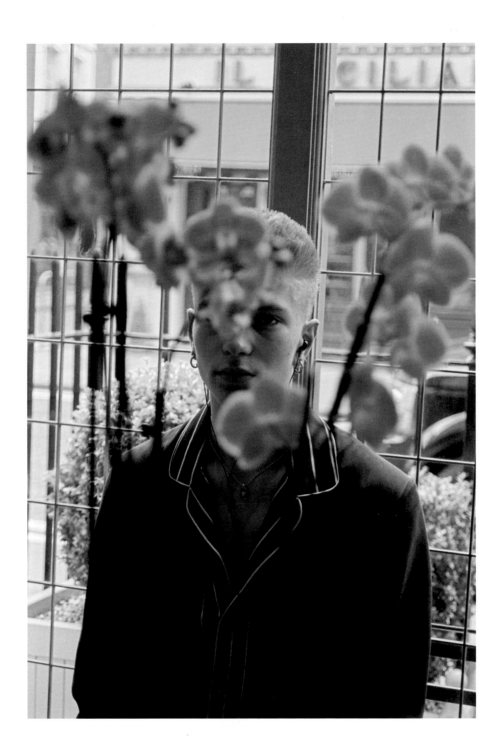

Bruna Kazinoti

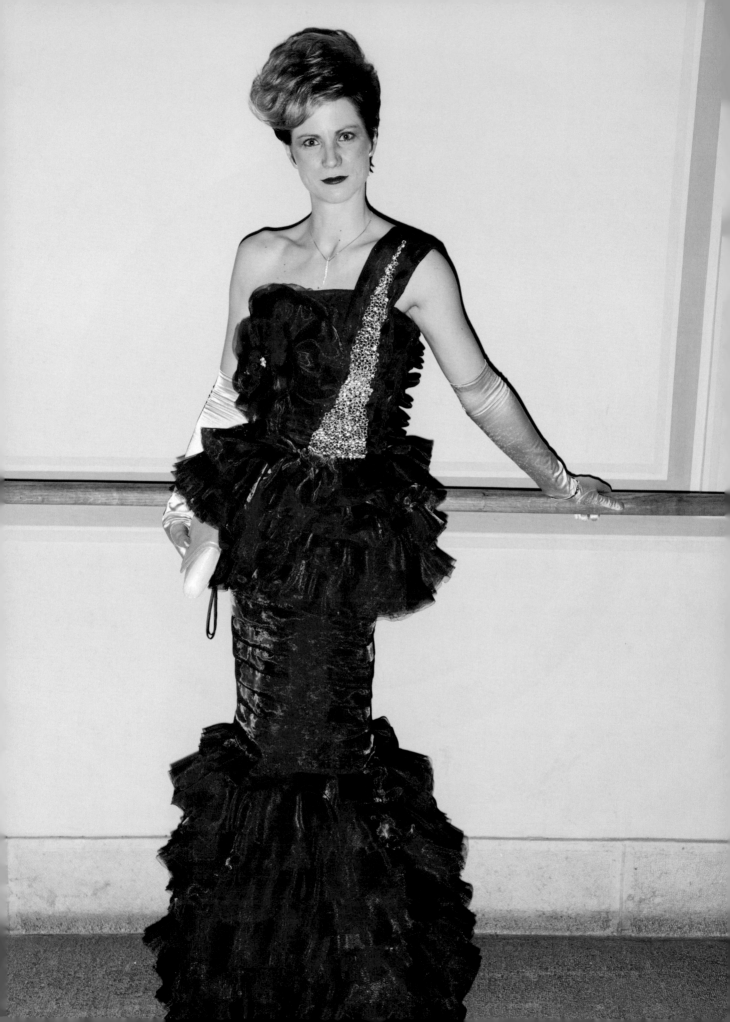

Immo Klink's extraordinary creative hybridity defies traditional categorization.

Immo Klink

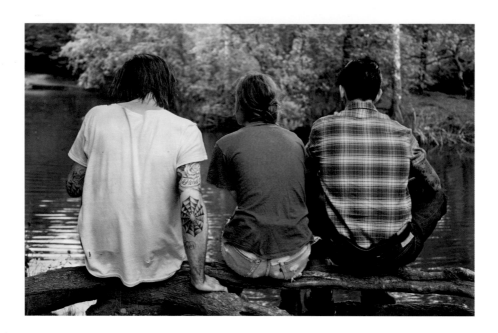

German photographer Immo Klink (b. 1972) is yet another new generation fashion image-maker whose extraordinary creative hybridity defies categorization. He did not follow the traditional route into the fashion industry: instead of undergoing formal photographic training and/or working for a prolonged period as a photographer's assistant, he read international law before moving to London in 1999 to commence further studies in intellectual property and business law. His master's degree politicized him, and his interest in multinational corporations and issues of globalization remains an important aspect of his photographic practice.

Klink worked in the London studio of Wolfgang Tillmans for a brief period in 2000, the year his fellow German was awarded the prestigious Turner Prize. The fluidity of Tillmans's approach, which spans fashion editorial, political documentary and more conceptual abstraction, with the photographer producing images for both magazine pages, and museum and gallery walls, had a formative influence on Klink.

Since starting out on his own, Klink has built up a substantial body of work, mostly using a 35 mm digital camera. In 2008, he began working with designer Miles Johnson on lookbooks for Levi's Vintage Clothing. The first project for Levi's, 'The Fall' for autumn/winter 2008, was based on his personal series on alternative European communities, a project that could be categorized as either social documentary or portraiture. In their examination of sub-cultural style and overall look, however, these earlier images could also be defined as fashion photographs (and some were in fact featured in *AnOther* magazine in 2006 under the editorship of Emma Reeves).

As advertising images, the Levi's photographs are necessarily more stylized in composition and dress. Models are depicted gathering wood and water, climbing trees, and standing in groups by lakes or in forests. Subsequent shoots for Levi's have ranged in style and theme, from 1930s boxers to 1950s bikers. Klink manipulates his images with techniques such as hand-dyeing and tinting, scratching and tearing, and he prints his pictures on alternative paper stocks. The final images are always unique and playful interpretations of the various collections.

A very different project was 'Vienna Opera Ball' for *Das Magazin* in 2011. As in most of his portrait work, Klink used a small hand-held camera with flash to create straightforward, realist snapshots. Thanks to his eye for incongruous detail and framing, the magazine reader is able to enter into a rarefied world of aristocratic privilege. Klink's images create layers of narrative and critique around promenade and performance, both documenting and deconstructing the elaborate gowns, jewels and hairstyles on display. Together, his single-frame colour portraits constitute a cleverly out-of-context 'post-fashion' story.

---

142 'Untitled 2' from 'Vienna Opera Ball', *Das Magazin*, 2011 — **144** 'Ozarks' for Levi's Vintage Clothing, 2009 — **145** 'Farewell' from *European Communities*, 2004
146 'Ladrón' from *European Communities*, 2003 — **147 left & right** 'Untitled 1' and 'Untitled 3' from 'Vienna Opera Ball', *Das Magazin*, 2011
148 above 'Dust&Wrath' for Levi's Vintage Clothing, S/S 2009 — **148 below** 'Boxer' for Levi's Vintage Clothing, 2012 — **149** 'The Fall' for Levi's Vintage Clothing, A/W 2008

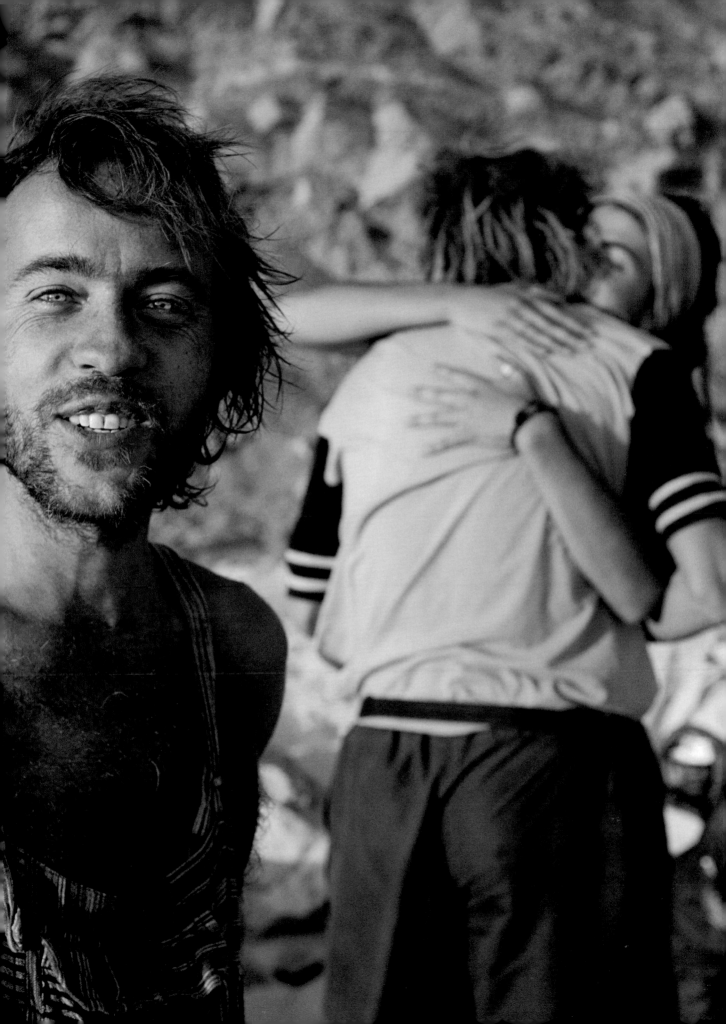

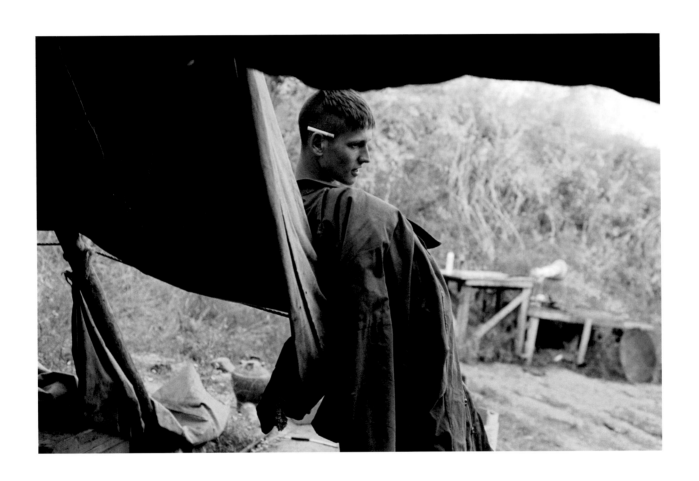

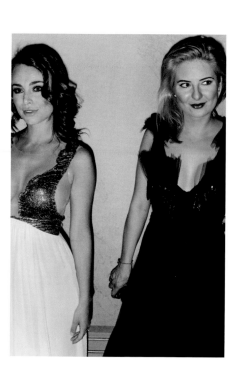

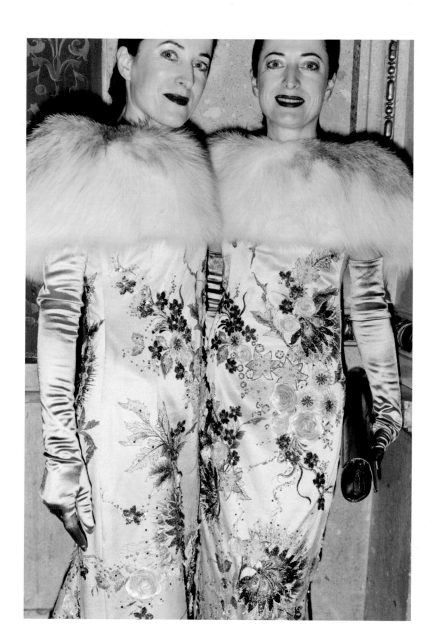

Immo Klink

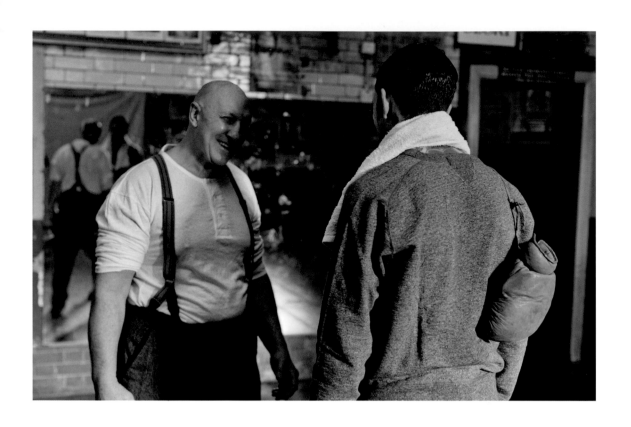

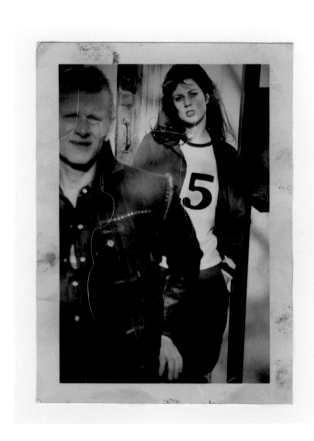

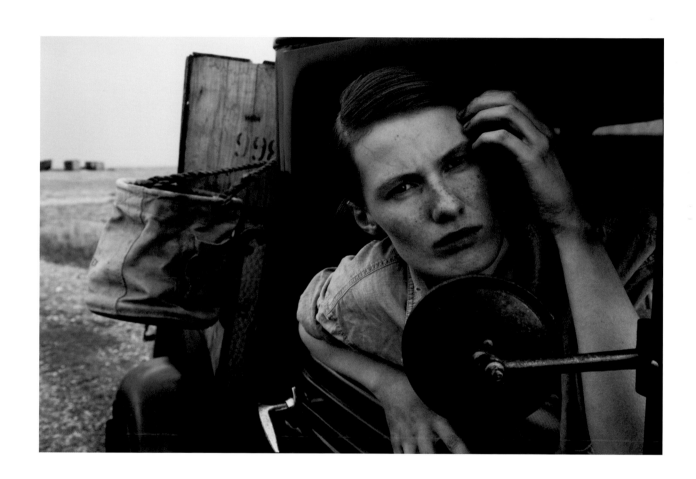

Immo Klink

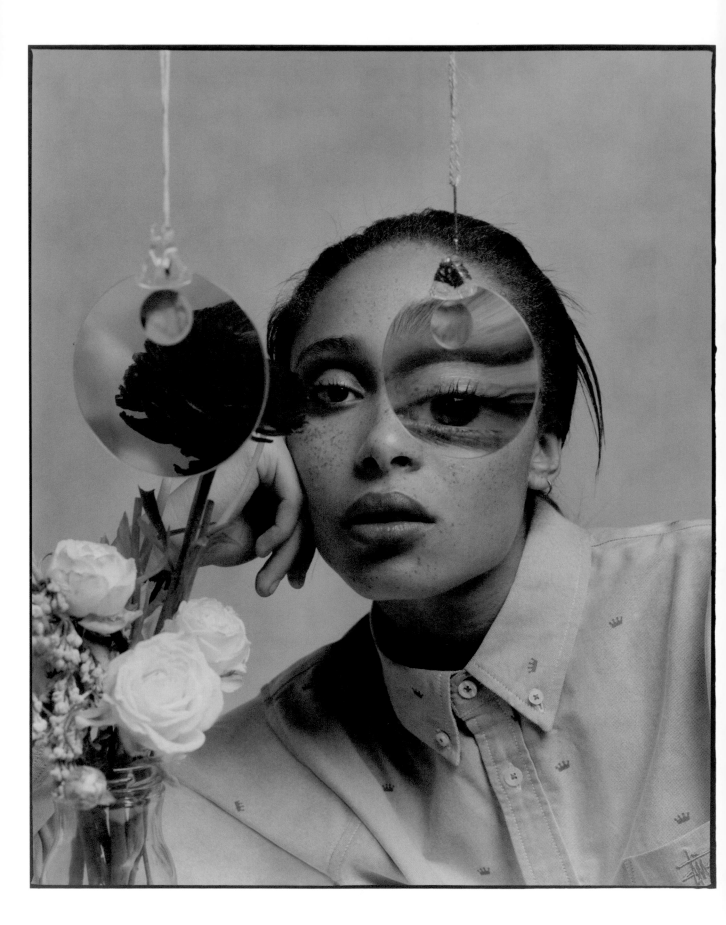

Tyrone Lebon's diverse and often collaborative practice embraces different media and experimental techniques.

Tyrone Lebon

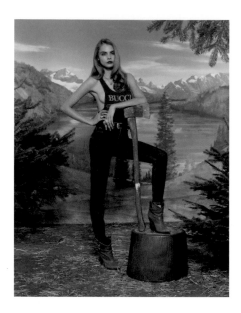

Like many artists with an uncompromising and distinctive creative voice, London-based photographer Tyrone Lebon (b. 1982) is inspired by the world around him – by his friends and family, his local hangouts, his favourite music, and the personal and social situations he finds himself in. Born in London, he is the son of the widely respected British fashion photographer Mark Lebon. Photography, which in Tyrone's case is a diverse and often collaborative process that continually embraces different media and experimental techniques, has been an inseparable part of his life since his teenage years.

Lebon began taking photographs at boarding school, making portraits of his friends and compiling them in dense visual diaries – a rough, cut-and-paste display format that he later adapted for his fashion editorials and advertising campaigns. This diaristic mode is evident in the photobook *Nothing Lasts Forever*, a collection of images of his friends and family that intentionally feel like fragments or snapshots rather than settled studio portraits. Published in 2011 by DoBeDo, an online collective founded by Lebon to provide a platform for emerging designers, photographers and filmmakers, the book is intimate and tender yet unapologetically resistant – to

sentimentality, to cultural and social stereotypes, and to offering a comfortable or easy description of the life experiences of its subjects.

After graduating from the University of Edinburgh with an MA in social anthropology in 2005, Lebon spent a period making documentary films. He soon received a commission from Terry Jones, the founding editor of *i-D*, which led to important collaborations with the magazine's former art director Dean Langley, and with Max Pearmain, a freelance stylist and the editor of *Arena Homme +*. Although he has produced editorials for many important fashion publications, working for *Pop* as well as *i-D* and *Arena Homme +*, Lebon is largely uninterested in constructing elaborate fashion narratives or in reinforcing mainstream ideals of beauty. His photographic process is unconventional: it is not uncommon for him to flaunt the rules of 'good' composition with techniques such as flare, overexposure, snapshot framing and cropping. For example, in 'Dancers Anon', a 2010 feature for Nike's *1948* magazine, Lebon includes the edges of the film reel in his photographs,

as though the images have come straight off the contact sheet. The studio setting, with its crumpled backdrop, is lo-fi, and although the dancers' poses are premeditated, their clothes – trainers, tops and tracksuits – are purely functional. Overall the images feel very uncontrived, an unusually relaxed and understated aesthetic that makes the story very relevant.

In a 2011 story for the Japanese magazine *Warp*, one of many collaborations with Pearmain, Lebon's brother Frank is pictured in clothes from the Supreme winter collection. The photographer himself appears in two of the images: we see his hand in the opening shot and later on his shadow. Once again, the fashion – in this case casual streetwear – is presented in the context of lived experience as Frank is photographed out and about in London. Although styled, the clothes are put through their paces in various real-life situations, including a trip to the dentist. A similar approach was used in another London-based collaboration with Pearmain: 'Alex / An Italian Mood' for *Arena Homme +*. Over the course of a month, Lebon documented the meanderings of the teenage Alex, who is always immaculately dressed in Italian tailoring and set apart from the unlikely goings on around him.

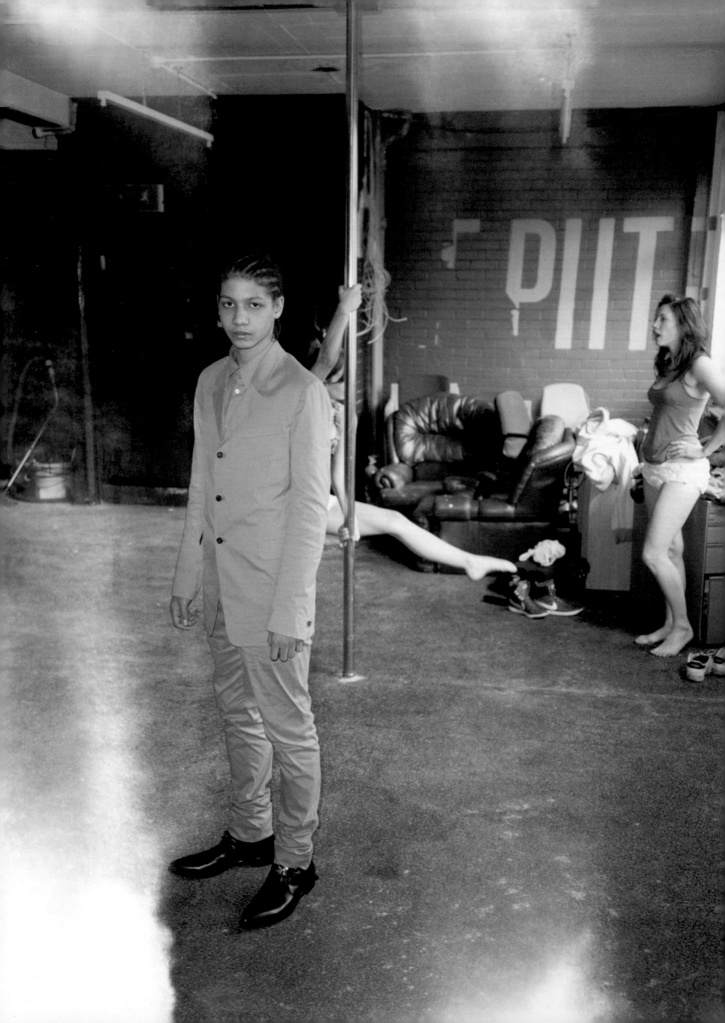

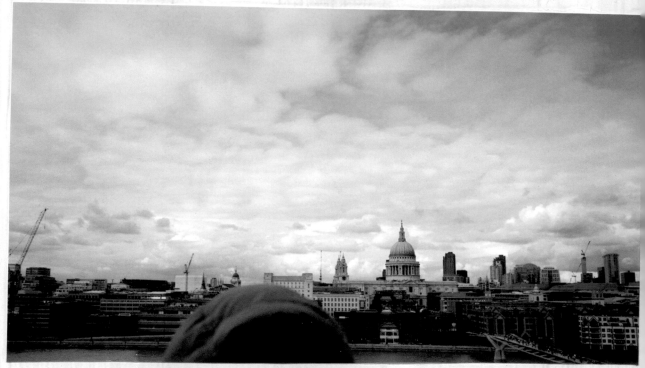
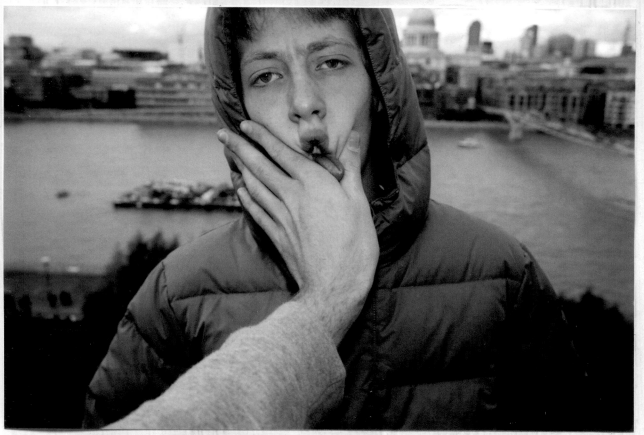

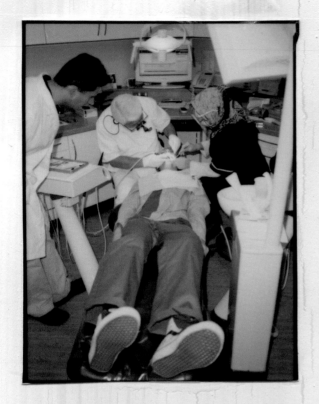
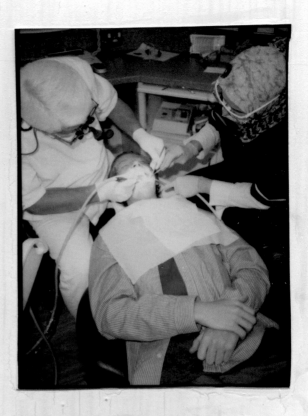
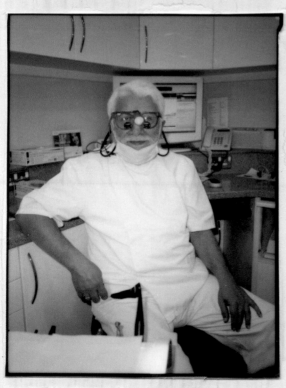
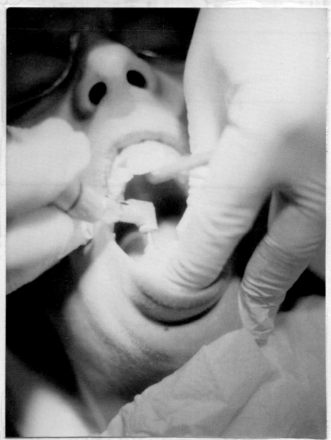

Tyrone Lebon

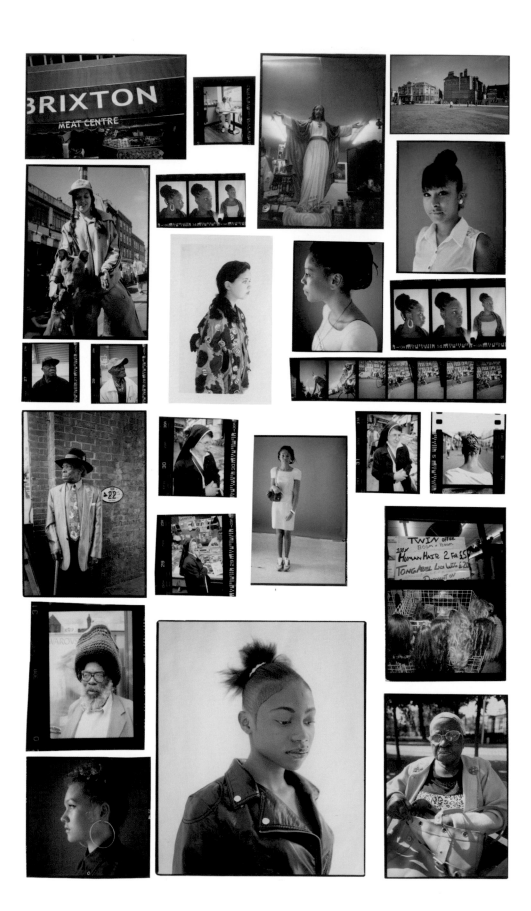

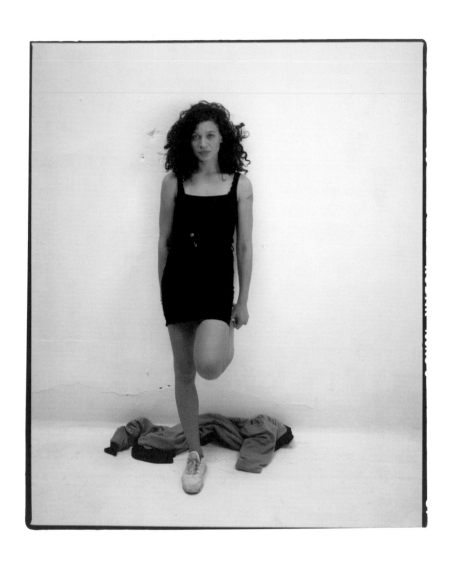

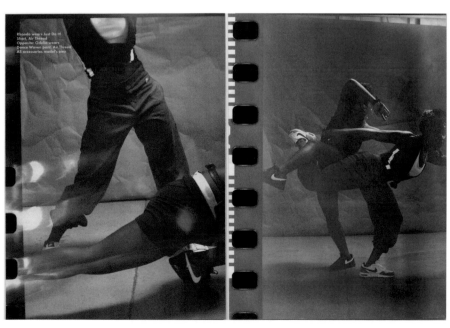

Rhonda wears Just Do It!
Short, Air Thread
Opposite: Odelia wears
Dance Woven pant, Air Thread
All accessories model's own

Tyrone Lebon

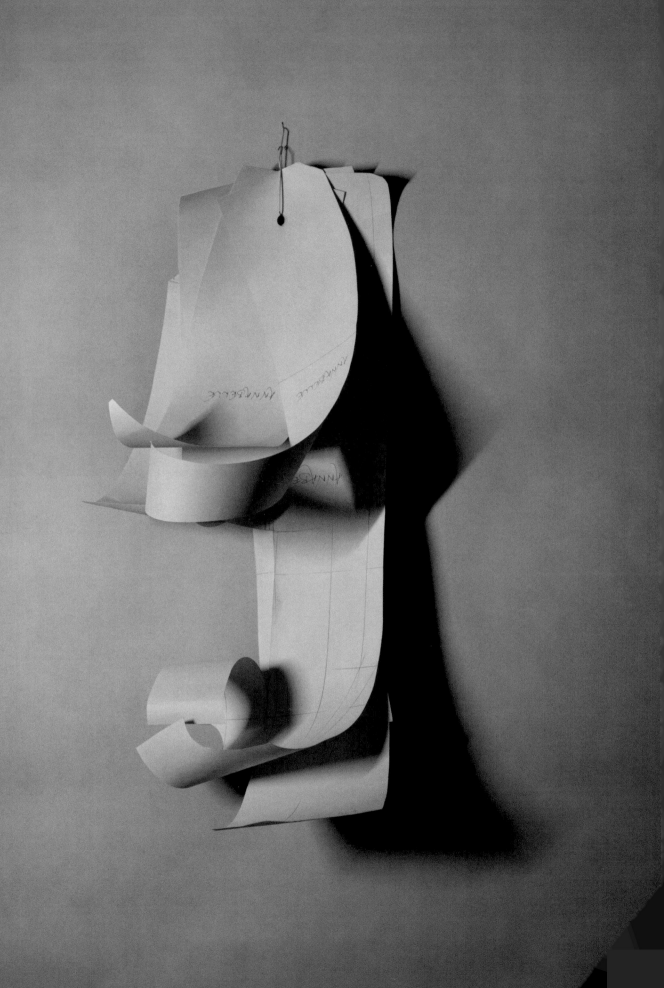

Joss McKinley's still-life tableaux often feature unexpected juxtapositions.

Joss McKinley

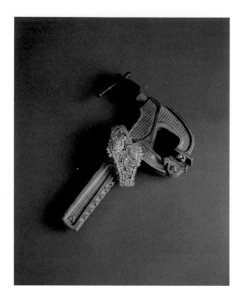

Joss McKinley (b. 1981) is a British photographer who lives and works between London and New York. He studied graphic design at Central Saint Martins College of Art and Design, discovering his affinity with photography in his foundation year. Working closely with design students on the menswear course, he made some early fashion images for the graduate catalogue in 2003, before embarking on an MA in fine-art photography at the London College of Communication. During the two-year course McKinley made *Underneath an Abject Window*, an important series that contains numerous compositional references to the historical tradition of *vanitas* painting. It is an early example of the painterly aesthetic that continues to define his still-life and fashion studies.

McKinley works mostly in film with large and medium-format cameras. Although he started out as a portrait photographer, he soon began creating still-life fashion stories. These clever tableaux are characterized by a careful arrangement of objects and often feature unexpected juxtapositions. For instance, in one

photograph from 'Rich Pickings', a 2012 story for *Telegraph Luxury*, a snail inches its way across diamond jewelry balanced on a rough granite rock, while in another a delicate gold necklace is strung across three bruised pears. In making these still lifes, McKinley is much less dependent on digital processes or elaborate artificial lighting than many of his contemporaries.

In 'Royal Warrant' for *enRoute* and 'Suits' for *Wallpaper**, the latter a beautifully balanced story about the construction of a Savile Row garment, McKinley is in his element. For both series, he photographed fashion items in simple settings – on a basic wooden table or against a plain, grey background – using light from a nearby window. We are welcomed into the photographer's working space, which is at once practical and fantastical. Each image features a single object – a bottle of scent, a box containing leather brogues, or a delicate blue coffee cup and teaspoon – with McKinley depicting these objects just as they are, but also transforming and ennobling them via the act of setting them apart. Many of his still-life photographs, such as 'Greens' for

Port magazine in 2012 or 'Soup' for the *Financial Times* in 2011, evoke the oddness and dead-end streets of Surrealist painting. Other projects – a 2013 gastronomy shoot for *Nowness*, for example, which documented the unusual collaboration between the Nordic Food Lab and Pestival, an international arts festival dedicated to insects – reveal his background in taxidermy (his father was a taxidermist) and interest in cycles of life and decay.

In 2010, McKinley worked with jeweller Hannah Martin and stylist Anders Soelvsten Thomsen on the fashion story 'The Man Who Knew Everything', using his skills as a portrait, landscape and still-life photographer to create a two-part narrative that combined very distinct styles and moods. His highly poetic, documentary-style series about interior reflection was the subject of the exhibition 'Gathering Wool' at Foam Fotografiemuseum Amsterdam in 2012. McKinley has also exhibited widely in the UK and his work can be found in numerous art collections, including the National Portrait Gallery and the University of the Arts Collection in London.

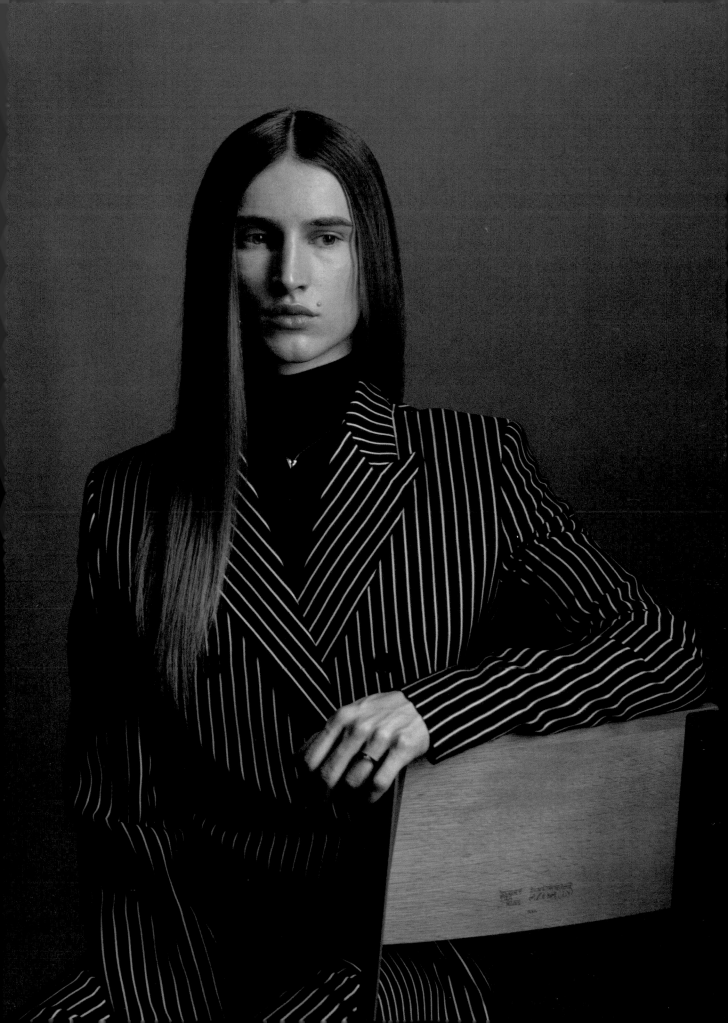

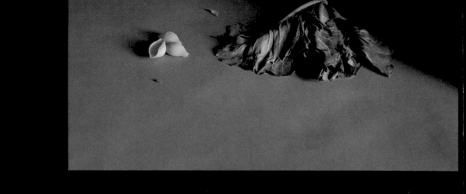
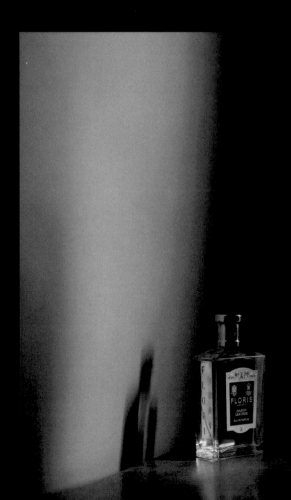

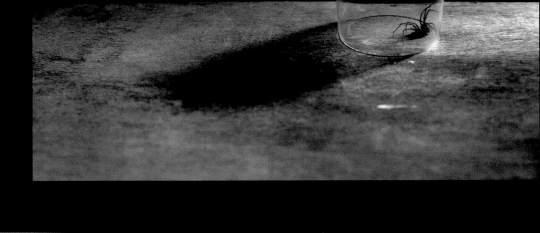

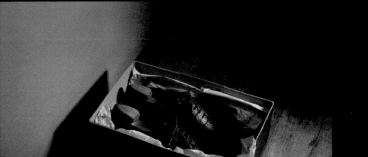

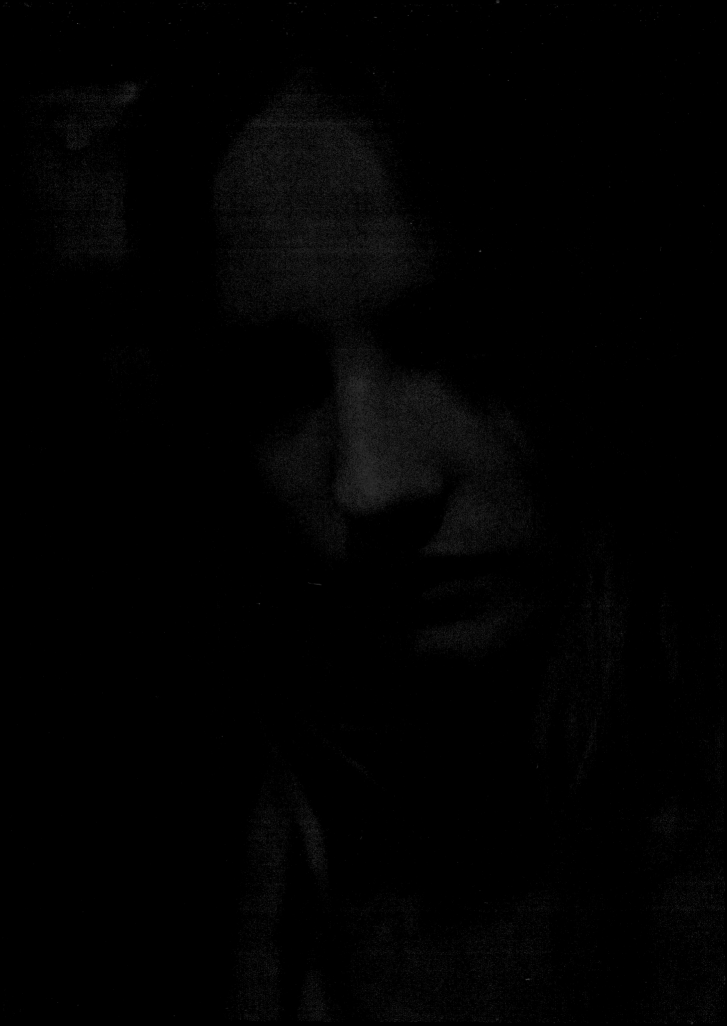

Chad Moore captures genuine reactions from his subjects while engaging with the parameters of fashion editorial.

Chad Moore

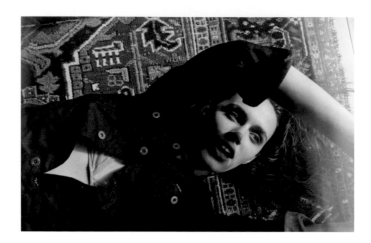

American photographer Chad Moore (b. 1987) grew up in Tampa, Florida. He was a successful BMX rider as an adolescent and began taking photographs of his friends cycling and doing tricks when he was about 14. Although he did eventually choose photography over bicycle-racing, he was put off by the highly technical and equipment-heavy approach of sports photography, disliking the need to prepare and predetermine – at least to some extent – the shots in advance and the staged look of much of the imagery.

In 2008, while partway through a business degree, Moore made a fortuitous move. He had just written off his car but instead of using the insurance money to buy a new one, he decided to quit his studies and follow a friend to New York, where he had always wanted to live. Upon arriving there he had no immediate plans, but he continued to take photographs, most often of his friends and the city night life and usually with Kyocera's Yashica T4. Intimate moments, group adventures and raucous parties – the youthful experiences of love, sex, ecstasy, sadness and pain – are relived in these raw and very visceral images. Later that year, Moore applied for an internship with American photographer

Ryan McGinley. To his surprise, his application was successful. In summer 2009, he accompanied McGinley and a crew of assistants and models on one of the acclaimed photographer's famous road trips across the USA. Since then, he has continued to assist McGinley while industriously pursuing his own projects. Despite his lack of formal training (except for the occasional high school and college class), he has managed to learn on the job and continues to test himself as new opportunities are presented.

Moore has been able to develop his own individual style, unshackled by the need to attain the 'correct' exposure, shutter speed or composition. He dislikes hard flash and has jokingly referred to the 'bad' light in his pictures. Some of his experiments involve placing a plastic bag over the camera lens and pointing it directly at various light sources such as TV screens and even the sun. Consequently, the sole information on the negative is colour, as though every frame in the entire roll of film had a filter. Moore then rewinds the film into the canister with the leader left out and starts taking his photographs. The resulting images are the product of an in-camera montage process, a subtle double-exposure technique that creates an effect

somewhere between a light leak, aged film and digital post-production.

As he gains more experience and his understanding of the medium strengthens, Moore has retained his preference for photographing people he knows well. He says that it sometimes gets to the point where he can anticipate their movements. Many of his friends are models, however, meaning that he is often inadvertently able to work with professionals.

Recently, Moore has worked on a number of more commercial, fashion-related projects. He always tries to capture a genuine reaction from his subjects and has managed to find a way to record these natural responses while staying within the parameters of fashion editorial. He still prefers to shoot on film, although uses both digital and analogue cameras for commercial jobs, depending on the client. So far, his photographs have been published in magazines such as *AnOther* and *Dazed & Confused*, and in 2011 the independent Berlin-based publisher PogoBooks released a softcover of his work entitled *Between Us*. Collections of his images have also been published by the German photography platform *dienacht* and the New York-based online gallery Glassine Box.

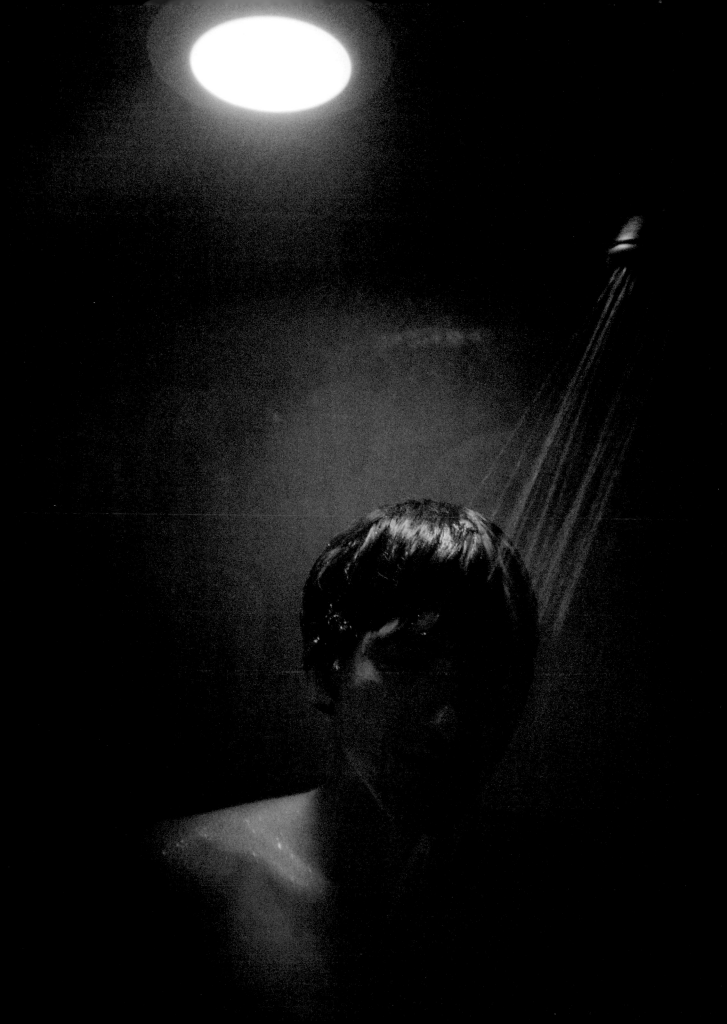

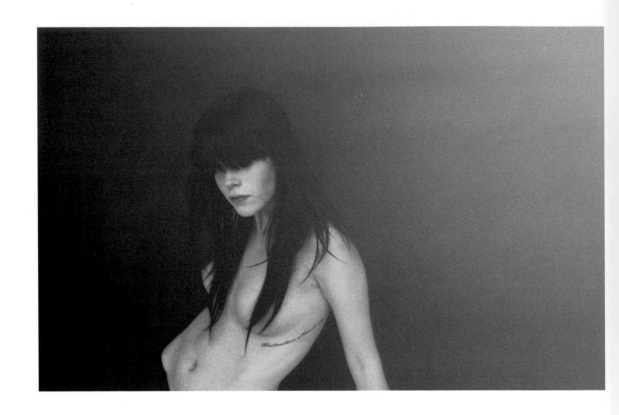

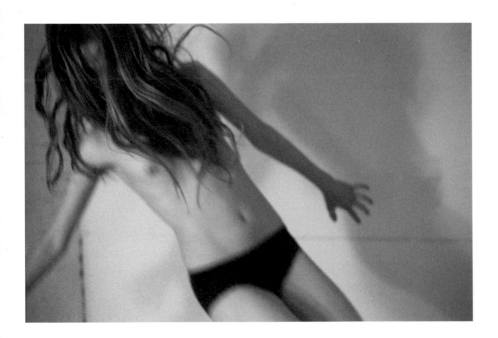

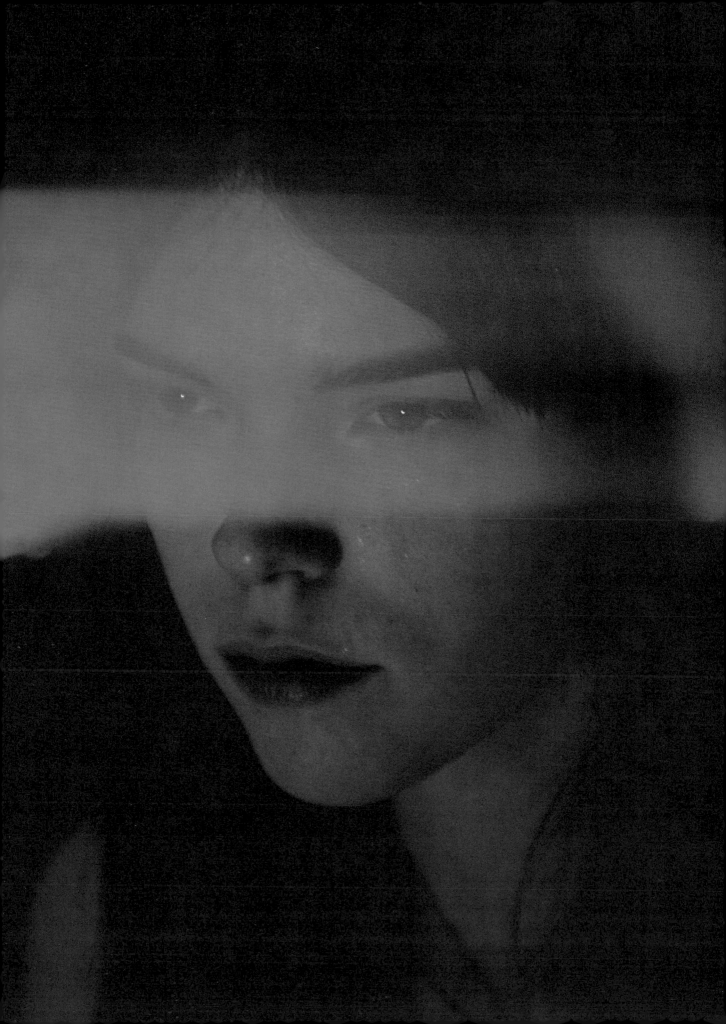

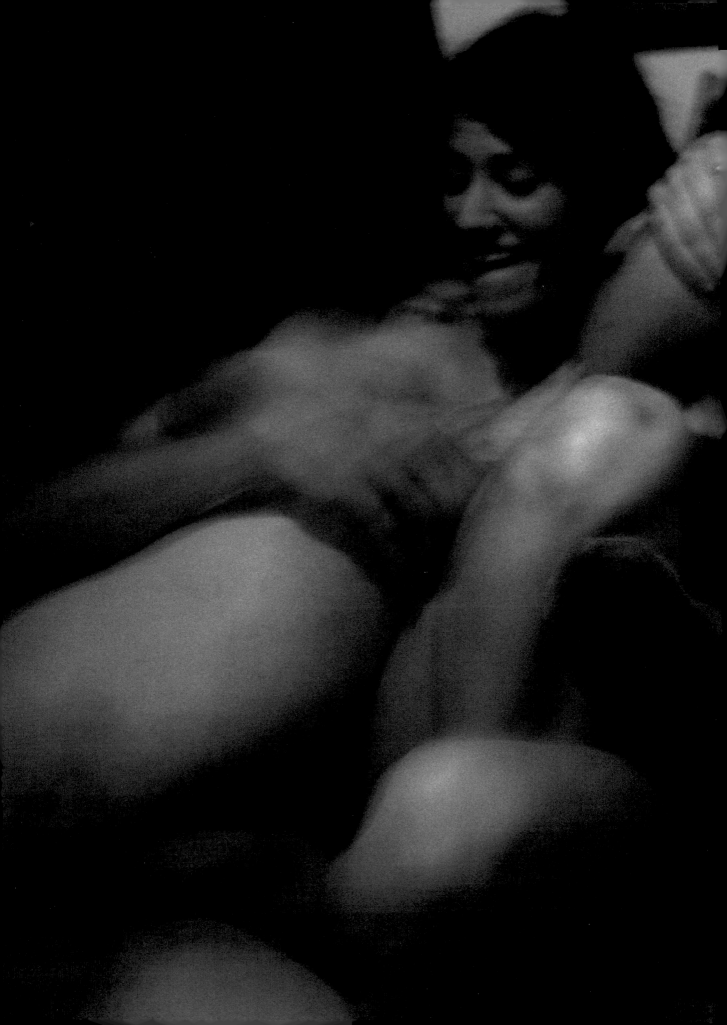

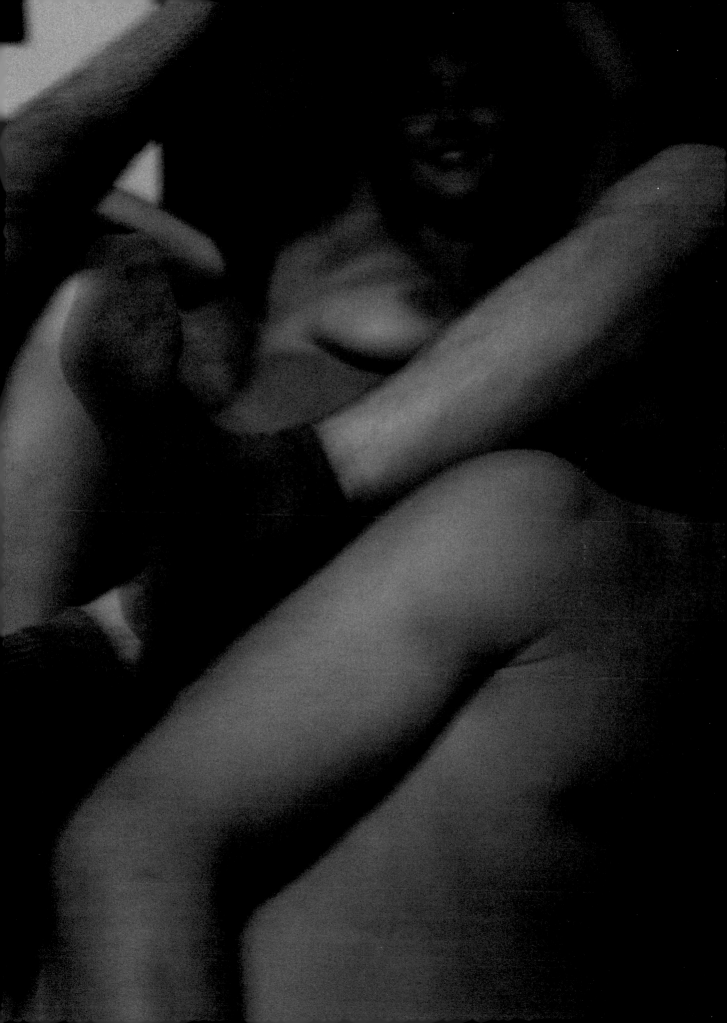

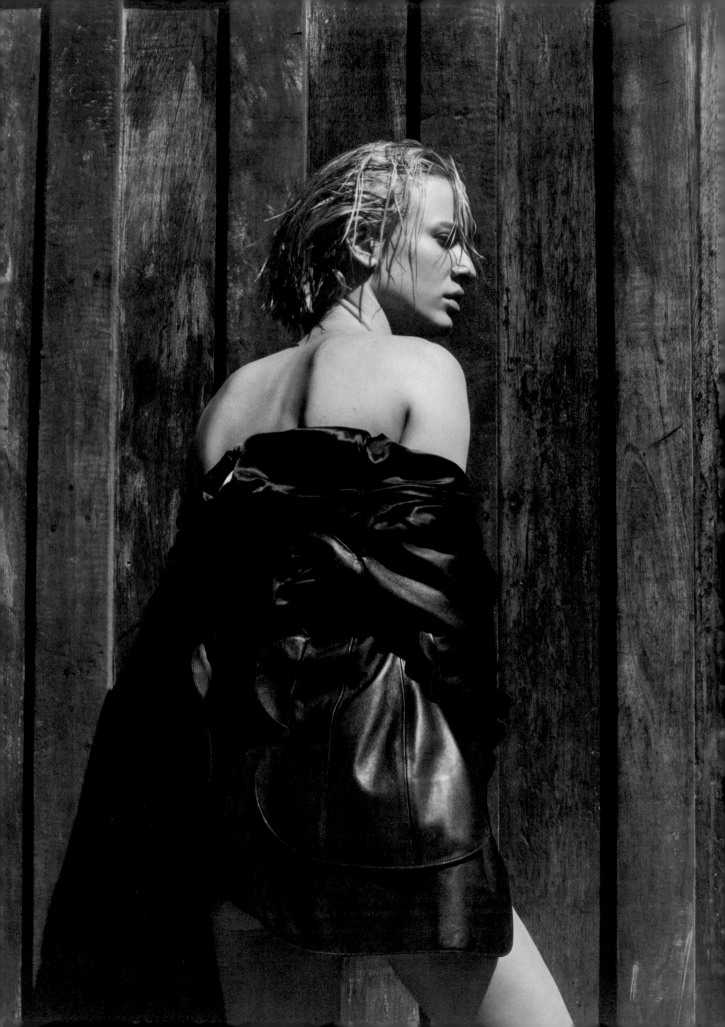

Laetitia Negre orchestrates shapes and poses that convey a sense of intimacy and power.

Laetitia Negre

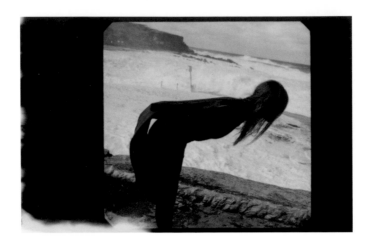

Laetitia Negre (b. 1975) is a French photographer who lives in London. She graduated from the University of Westminster with a BA in film, video and photographic arts in 1999. After working for a brief period as a runner on music videos, Negre moved into fashion photography. Her training was highly technical, and a very precise control of her favoured apparatus (medium and large-format film cameras) and lighting remains central to her practice.

Negre uses Polaroid creatively in her fashion editorials, combining the one-offs with images made from film negatives. Traditionally, Polaroids were the first images made on set before the photographer began to expose the film. Prior to the advent of digital technology, which enables photographers to see the shots instantaneously on a computer screen, Polaroids were used to experiment with lighting and compositional alternatives and to test out different outfits, hairstyles and makeup. Unlike digital fashion photographs, which are often highly retouched and almost impossibly flawless, Polaroids have a distinct quality of imperfection.

Negre's astute awareness of the potential of Polaroid to elicit a very different kind of relationship between model and photographer is a defining feature of her approach. 'Haute Couture', a 2010 story for *Zoo* magazine with Brazilian model Daiane Conterato, demonstrates the subtle shift in mood and intensity that occurs when these less formal images are displayed alongside more composed fashion photographs. In the Polaroids, the distance between photographer and subject is collapsed: Negre's presence is much more obvious than in the 'clean' images, where it is singularly Conterato who is the subject of the pictures.

Another important aspect of Negre's work is the mutual understanding that exists between her and her subjects, who are usually women. As a result, her photographs are often celebratory representations of female physicality, with an emphasis on individual authority rather than submissive sexuality. This is brilliantly achieved in two separate editorials for *Zoo*, one with Romanian model Diana Dondoe and another with Australian model Emma Balfour. In photographing these relatively simple studio portraits Negre worked much

like a choreographer, directing the models' shapes and poses so as to convey a sense of intimacy and power. The inclusion of Polaroids in the Balfour story, which was shot on location in Australia, brings us closer to Negre herself, drawing our attention to her directorial role in the picture-making process.

We witness Negre's ability to translate dynamic movement into still sculptural form at exactly the right moment in the 2011 project 'Raw', which features Romanian-Canadian model Irina Lăzăreanu in a number of statement poses against a plain, white background. The elegance of Negre's direction and her intelligence in the studio is also evident in 'Ready 2 Be', a 2012 editorial for *D – la Repubblica* magazine with stylist Davide Brambilla. Here, she photographed models in three-quarter length against a white backdrop, creating a series of striking colour and compositional contrasts across the editorial sequence between the white-on-white and black-on-white images.

---

172 'My Pretty Seahorse', *i-D*, 2009 — **174** Emma Balfour, *Zoo*, 2011 — **175** Diana Dondoe, *Zoo*, 2011
176 left 'Raw', 2011 — **176 right** 'Ready 2 Be', *D – la Repubblica*, 2012 — **177 above & centre** 'Haute Couture', *Zoo*, 2010
177 below 'Ready 2 Be', *D – la Repubblica*, 2012

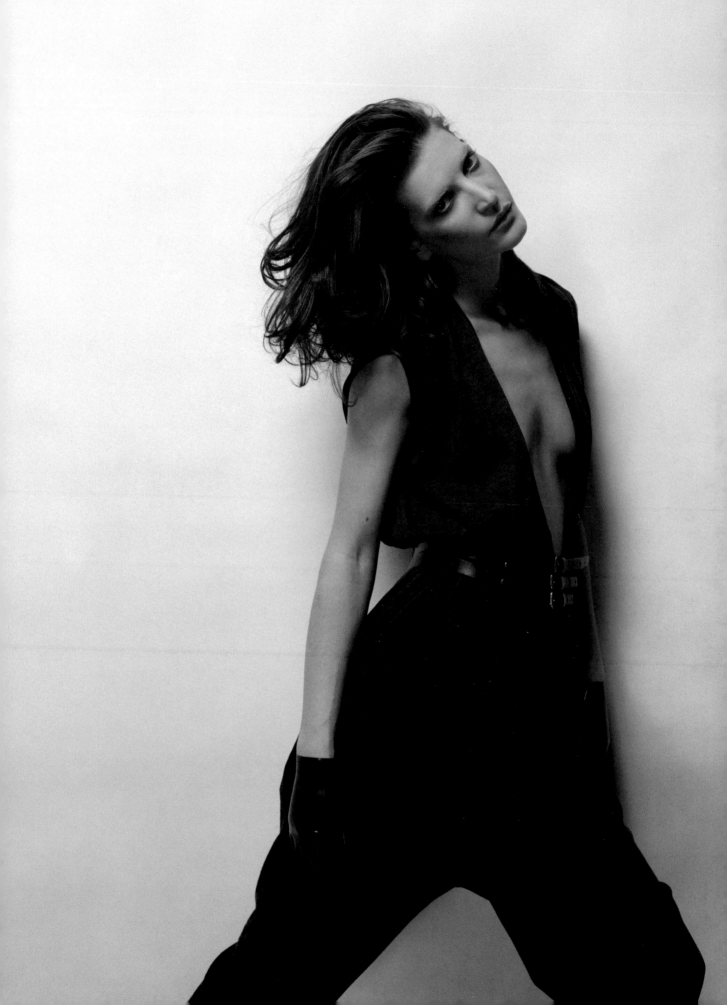

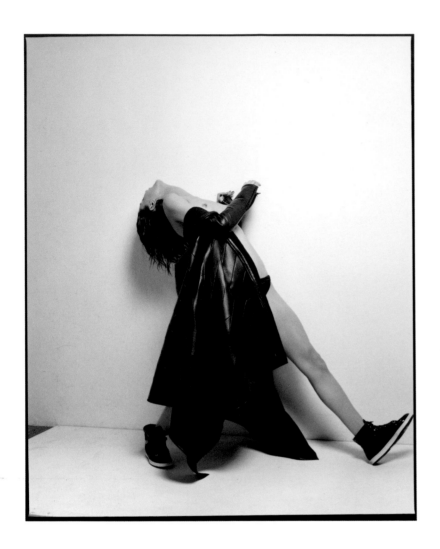

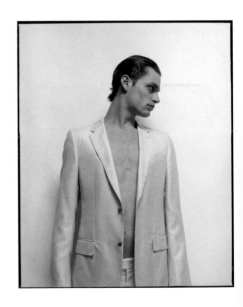

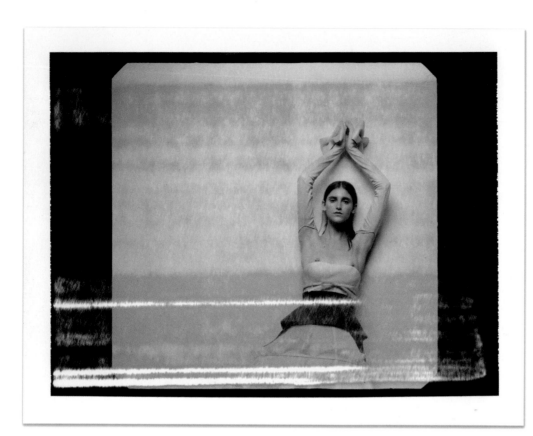

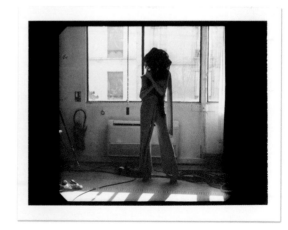

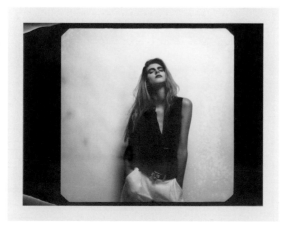

Laetitia Negre

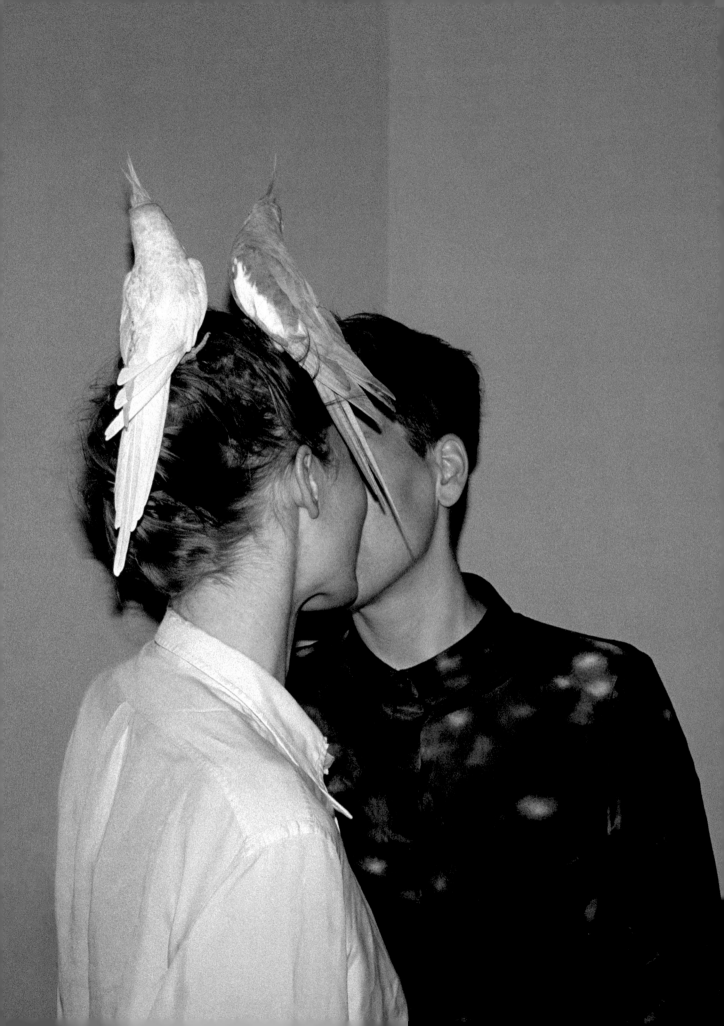

Hanna Putz is interested in formal aspects of image-making such as colour contrasts and the relations between objects.

Hanna Putz

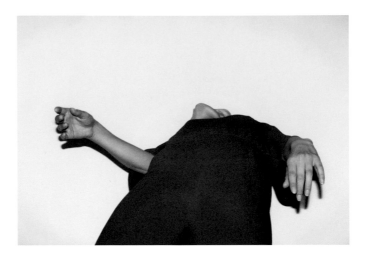

Hanna Putz (b. 1987) is an Austrian photographer based in London. She worked as a model for seven years before concentrating exclusively on photography, which had always been a hobby. Apart from the occasional pieces of advice from the photographers she modelled for, Putz is self taught. In her approach to photography, however, she demonstrates a maturity and rigour well beyond her years.

Although she has worked in the fashion industry for some time, Putz does not consider herself to be a fashion photographer. Instead, she describes herself as a photographer who occasionally shoots fashion, but prefers to take pictures of people she knows well. Although her images often feature professional models, this is merely a by-product of her previous career as many of these models are her friends. Putz wants her subjects to feel at ease and unselfconscious in front of her lens, explaining why most of her images are set in private or domestic spaces, where people tend to be more comfortable.

Putz is more interested in the formal aspects of image-making – in colour contrasts and the relations between objects, and in the way her subjects pose and interact with their surroundings – than in the technical side of the medium. She works exclusively with film and usually with natural light. The resulting images are always stripped free of superfluous detail, with Putz preferring to shoot relatively minimal backgrounds, plain interiors and unpatterned clothes.

For a 2012 series published in *New York* magazine, Putz was given a number of monochrome pieces by the magazine's fashion editor to photograph as she liked. In one image, a woman in a blue dress stands with her back to us, holding a baby on her shoulders in such a way that we are unable to see her head. Only the woman's slender arm is visible as it extends up above her head and curls round the child's back, creating a beautiful symmetry between her elbow and the child's bent arm. This photograph is a perfect example of the way Putz treats her fashion editorials: she makes the images she wants of the people who interest her in contexts that are suggestive of their personality. In this way, the fashion elements become almost an aside.

Putz's particular approach requires a lot of freedom and trust from her publishers.

Rather than taking photographs for the sake of creating new editorials, with each project she aims to refine her personal vision. She tries to make images that force us to consider the way her subjects' poses, gestures, identities and attitudes can be captured, questioned and even generated by the camera lens.

It is no surprise, then, that Putz admires the work of Roni Horn, Rineke Dijkstra, Taryn Simon and Philip-Lorca diCorcia, all of whom have covered significant ground in portrait and/or conceptual photography. In 2012, she was one of ten finalists at the International Festival of Fashion and Photography in Hyères. Besides France, she has exhibited her work in Austria, Germany, Cyprus, the USA and the UK, where her photographs of mothers and daughters were some of the highlights of Susan Bright's exhibition 'Home Truths: Photography, Motherhood and Identity' at the Photographers' Gallery in London in 2013. Putz's images have also appeared in numerous publications, including *Zeitmagazin*, *Dazed & Confused*, *Husk*, *Tissue* and *Under/Current*, among others. She continues to work on exhibitions and personal projects.

---

178 'Untitled (Grand 2)', 2012 — 180 'Untitled (De Wavrin 1)', *Oyster*, 2012 — 181 'Stand der Dinge', *New York*, 2012
182 above 'Untitled (A.M.1)' from *Untitled 2011–2013*, 2011 — 182 below 'Untitled (MV 1)', *New York*, 2012
183 'Untitled (LL 1)', *New York*, 2012

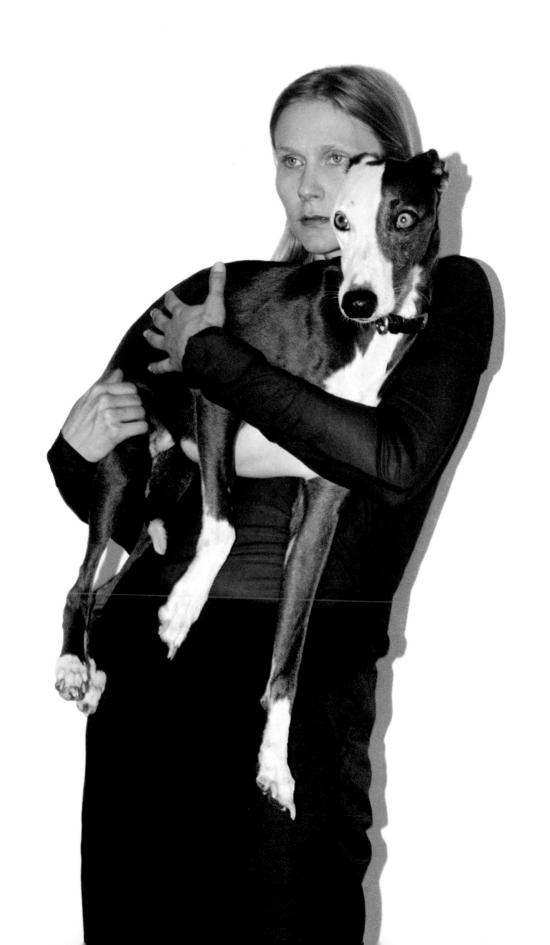

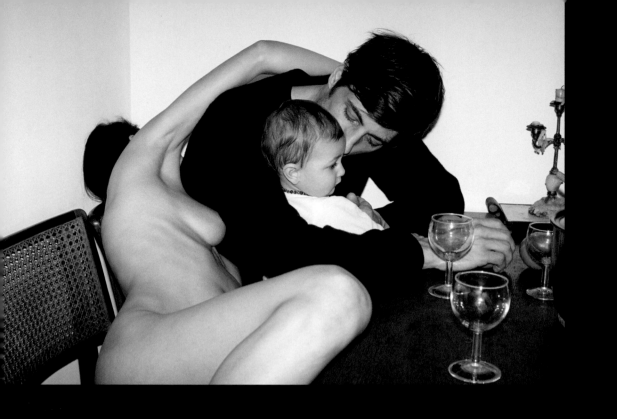

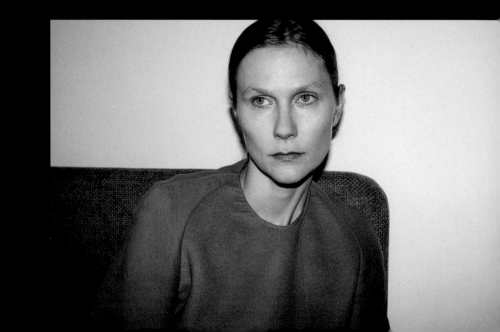

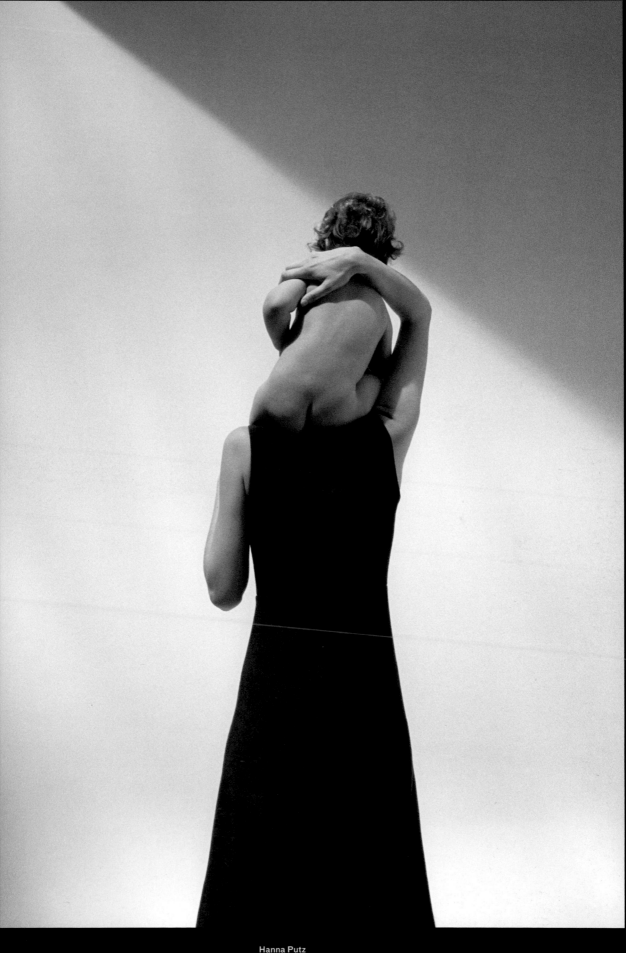

Hanna Putz

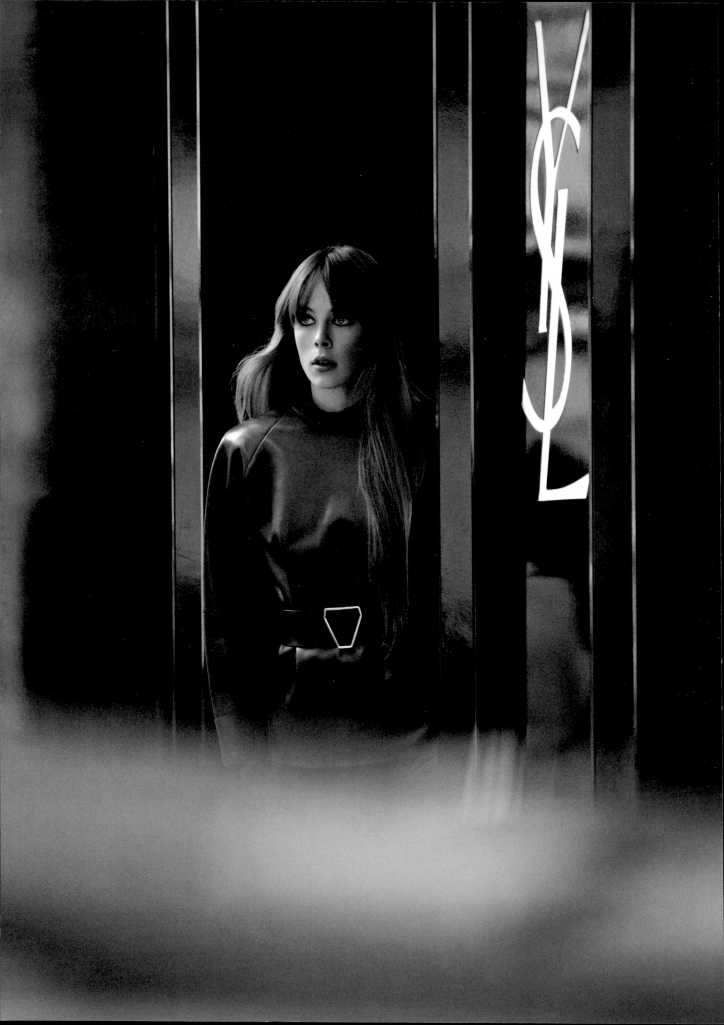

Daniel Riera's position is often that of the unobserved voyeur: his models appear to be unaware of his camera lens.

Daniel Riera

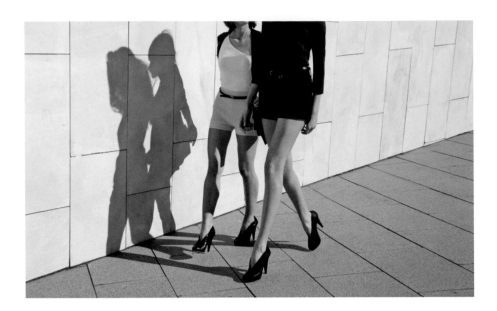

Daniel Riera (b. 1970) is a Spanish photographer who lives and works between London and Barcelona. He studied fine art and photography at the University of Barcelona and cinema at the Escola De Mitjans Audovisuals, also in Barcelona. As a student, he lived across the road from a cinema and was an avid filmgoer; his decision to become a professional photographer and subsequent aesthetic were shaped as much by his interest in cinema and the moving image as by his formal photographic training. He began working in the late 1990s, making portraits and CD covers for independent Spanish magazines such as *aB*, *Disco 2000*, *b-guided*, *Neo2* and *Vanidad*. During this time of creative freedom, he was introduced to the stylist Oscar Visitación, marking the start of an important working relationship.

At the beginning of his career, Riera shot exclusively on film, using medium-format cameras as well as a hand-held Leica 35 mm. He now works digitally, although since losing all his equipment at a Cuban airport he has placed less emphasis on his cameras. Instead, he relies on impulse to capture a particular mood or expression. Portrait sequences for the magazines *Electric Youth!* and *Hercules* employ an energetic and highly personal documentary style. These playful black-and-white images flaunt the rules of 'correct' technique, conveying a sense of spontaneity and intimacy.

In the mid-2000s, the Dutch magazine designer, editor and publisher Jop van Bennekom asked Riera to shoot fashion features for *Butt*. Riera soon began to work for a newer crop of less glossy, more intelligent publications, including Penny Martin's *The Gentlewoman* and *Fantastic Man*, another of van Bennekom's projects. In these more recent editorials, Riera's position is that of the unobserved voyeur. He tends to shoot outdoors, often on city streets, where his models go about their business seemingly unaware of the camera lens. For example, in 'City Suits', a *Fantastic Man* editorial shot on location in New York in 2011, a suited businessman purposefully carries his dry cleaning home, oblivious to the existence of the photographer. Elsewhere, in the cinematographic, suspense-laden story 'Y Tu Mamá También', which appeared in Spanish *V* in 2011, Dafne Cejas plays a female torero absorbed in the moment before her performance. Riera was an unobtrusive presence yet again in two stories published in *The Gentlewoman* in 2012: in 'Electricity', where Julia Nobis was captured running across a barren landscape populated only by wind turbines; and 'Ready to Wear Right Now', which featured Edie Campbell as a glamorous girl about town frequenting the best Parisian boutiques.

In another strand of his work, Riera demonstrates his flair for composition by dramatically cropping photographs to highlight a particular garment. When seen over a number of pages, these crops of apparel such as shoes or trousers become poignant narrative details suggesting an accident or a fetishistic moment that was not meant to be photographed.

—

184 'Ready to Wear Right Now with Edie Campbell', *The Gentlewoman*, 2012 — 186 'Tall 'N' Small', *The Gentlewoman*, 2010
187 'Y Tu Mamá También', *V* (Spain), 2011 — 188 'Youssef, Assilah' — 189 above 'City Suits', *Fantastic Man*, 2011
189 below 'Vacation', *Fantastic Man*, 2012 — 190–191 'Electricity', *The Gentlewoman*, 2012

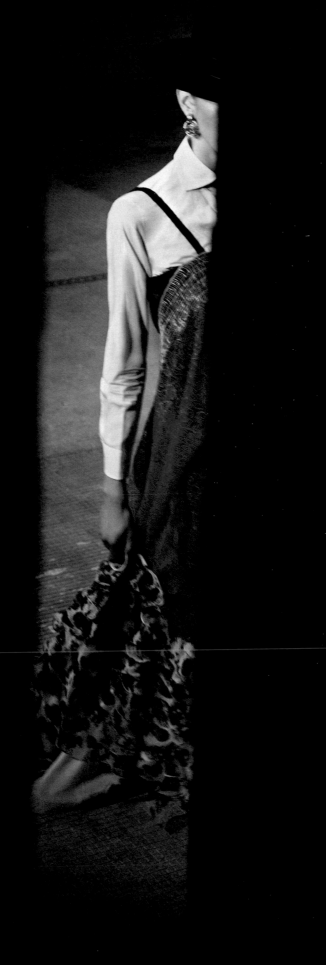

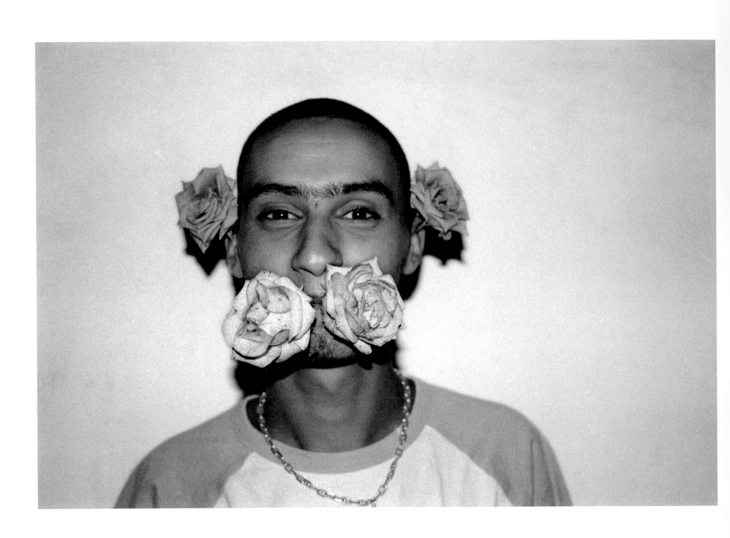

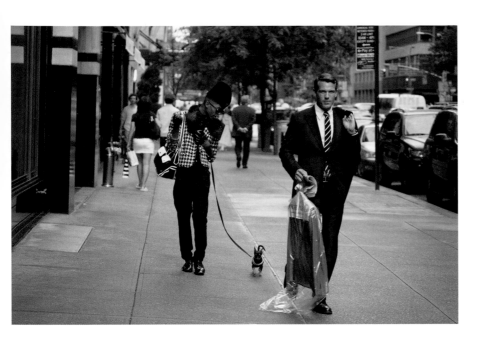

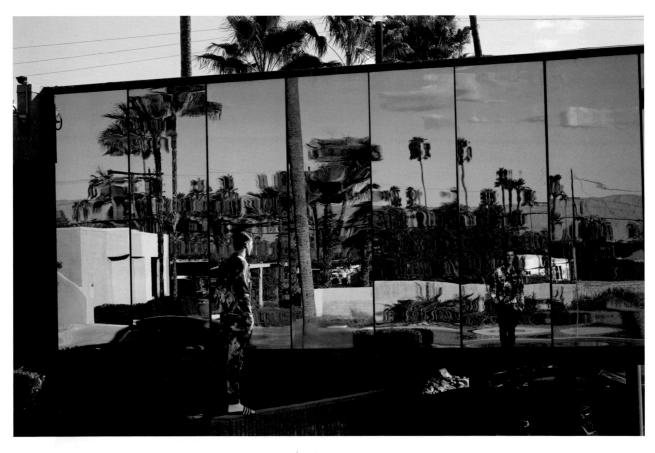

Daniel Riera

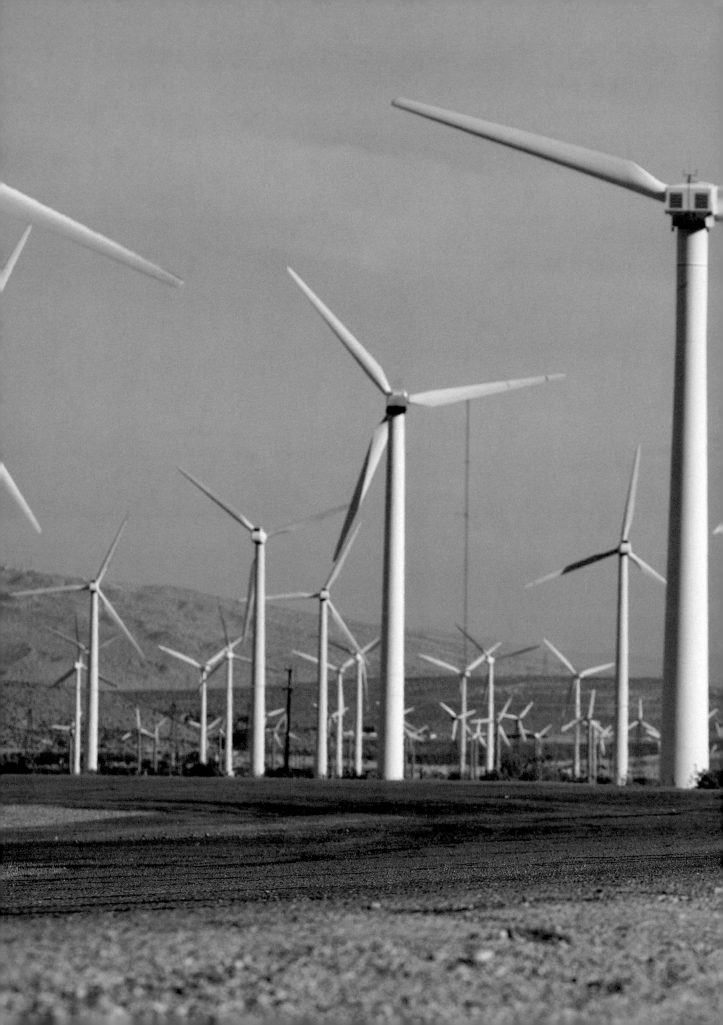

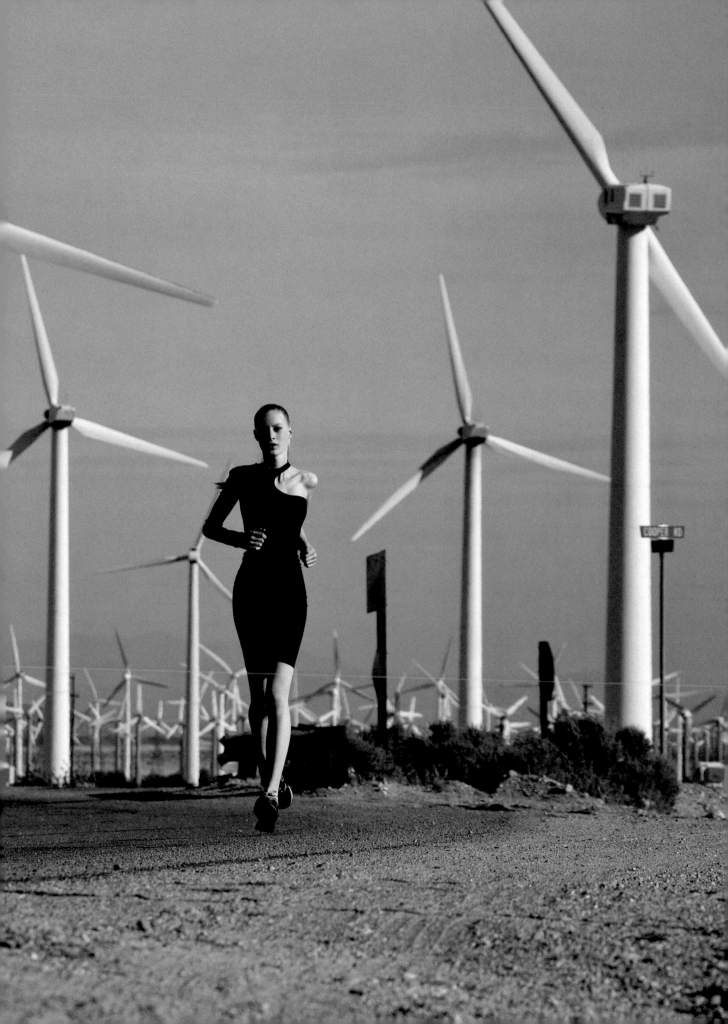

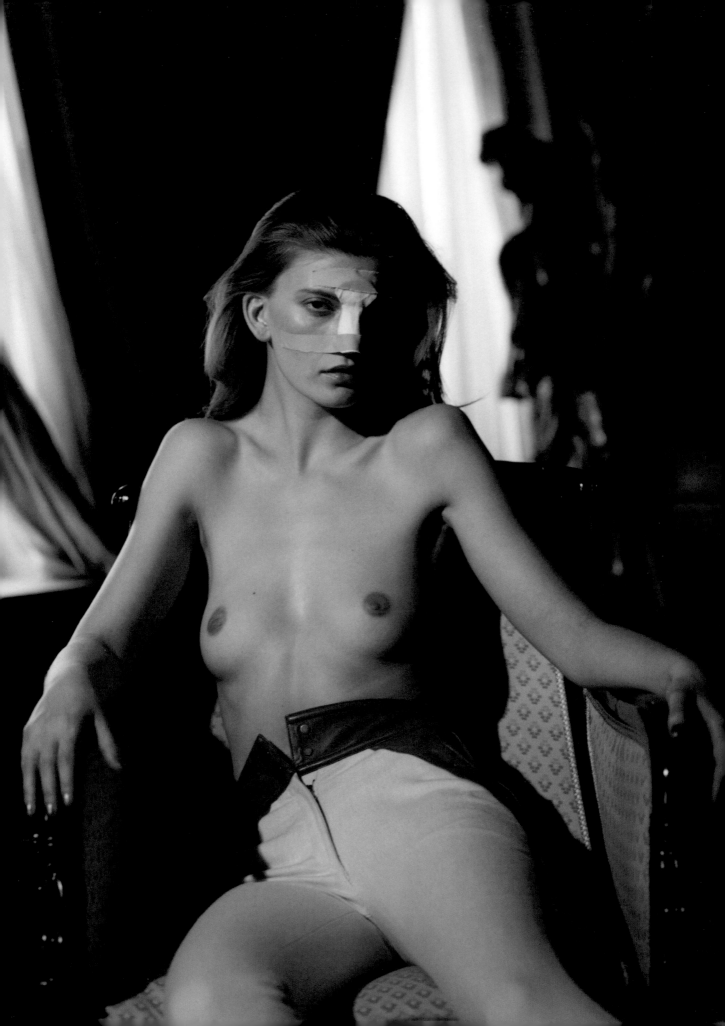

Robi Rodriguez works like a film director or novelist, developing stories that unfold gradually.

Robi Rodriguez

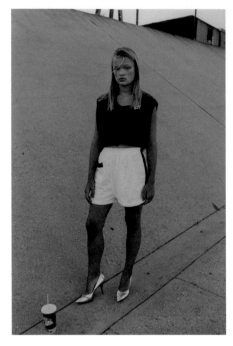

Robi Rodriguez (b. 1972) is a Spanish photographer who lives and works in London. He began taking photographs at the age of 27 while studying film at the Art Center College of Design in Pasadena, California. It was at an Art Center lecture that Rodriguez met the controversial but hugely influential American photographer Bob Richardson, who offered him the opportunity to work as an assistant.

Rodriguez's creative process is highly considered, beginning with a narrative concept and involving a careful orchestration of lighting, movement and setting. He works like a film director or novelist, developing characters and scenarios that evolve and unfold gradually over the whole image sequence.

In early straight-ups taken in Los Angeles soon after he finished assisting, Rodriguez experimented with creating strong characters. By deliberately photographing his models in nondescript urban settings against stark concrete backgrounds and with only natural light, he challenged himself to convey depth and personality. The resulting images rely on their subjects' individual sense of style, as well as Rodriguez's sensitivity and his intuitive timing as a photographer to capture a transformative pose or expression.

Like several of the photographers in this book, Rodriguez has exhibited his work at the International Festival of Fashion and Photography in Hyères, an important platform for emerging practitioners of the genre. In 2006 he showed his series *The Birds*, a personal project about the emotionally complex relationship between a late middle-aged couple. In its intensity and intimacy, this story remains one of his most powerful works.

Fashion plays an important part in other personal projects about human, and especially sibling, relationships. *Unlimited Love*, for example, was a series of portraits of Rodriguez's two adopted sisters taken between 2007 and 2009. He styled the young girls himself, often in adult garments, so that fashion remains a constant in the otherwise ambiguous tableaux. Similarly, the 2011 story *Curiel* was about three sisters related to Rodriguez's family. Here, the uniformity of the women's clothes, jewelry and set hairstyles across the image sequence creates a narrative tension that underpins the photographer's exploration of the sisters' different personalities.

'Bad Moon Rising', the most memorable story in *Pop* magazine's spring/summer 2012 issue, was a modern-day, *King Kong*-esque love saga in which a beautiful girl and a gorilla played out a sexually charged domestic drama. In the photographs, the high-fashion garments worn by Slovenian model Valerija Kelava function as mechanisms of power and seduction. And yet the fetishistic pretence of this is underscored by the absurdity of the situation: the girl is dressing for an ape, and an obviously fake one at that. The gorilla is both a semi-tragic character – a misunderstood outsider who inspires sympathy – and a figure of ridicule. One image, where Kelava sits, hands placed demurely in her lap, with the ape crouching fearsomely by her side, is a pastiche of the formal studio 'couples' portrait. Superbly styled by Vanessa Reid, this confident, adventurous and playful fashion story is a great example of the ingenious ability of Rodriguez – and many other new generation photographers – to present seriously good fashion while working outside the narrative constructs traditionally associated with fashion photography.

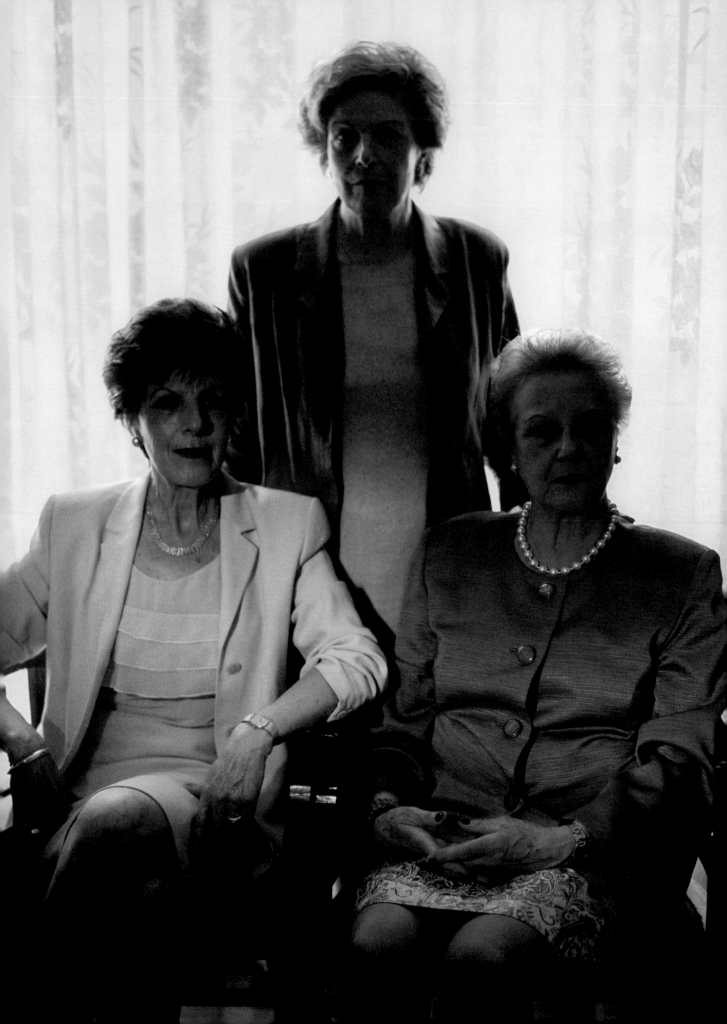

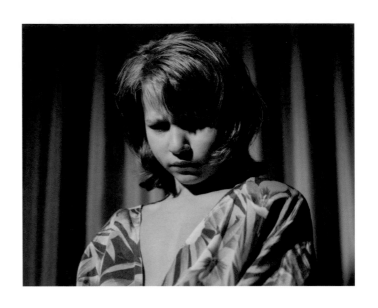

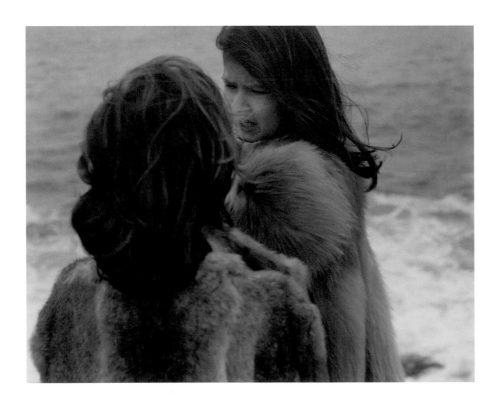

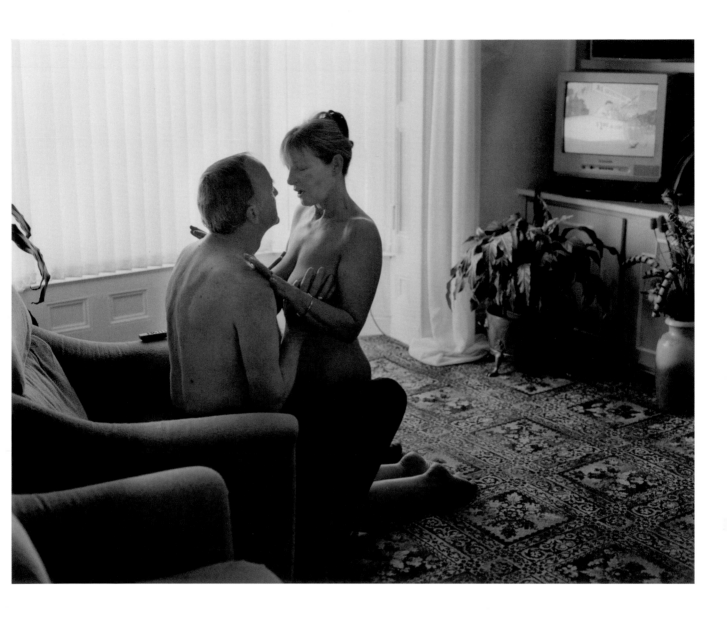

Robi Rodriguez

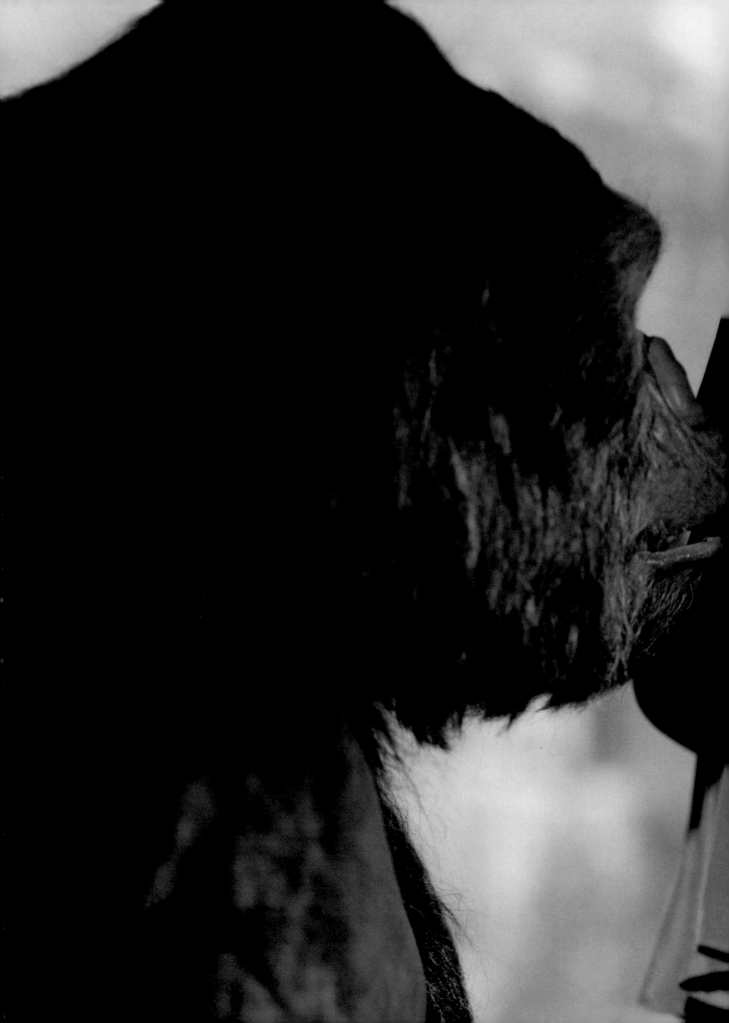

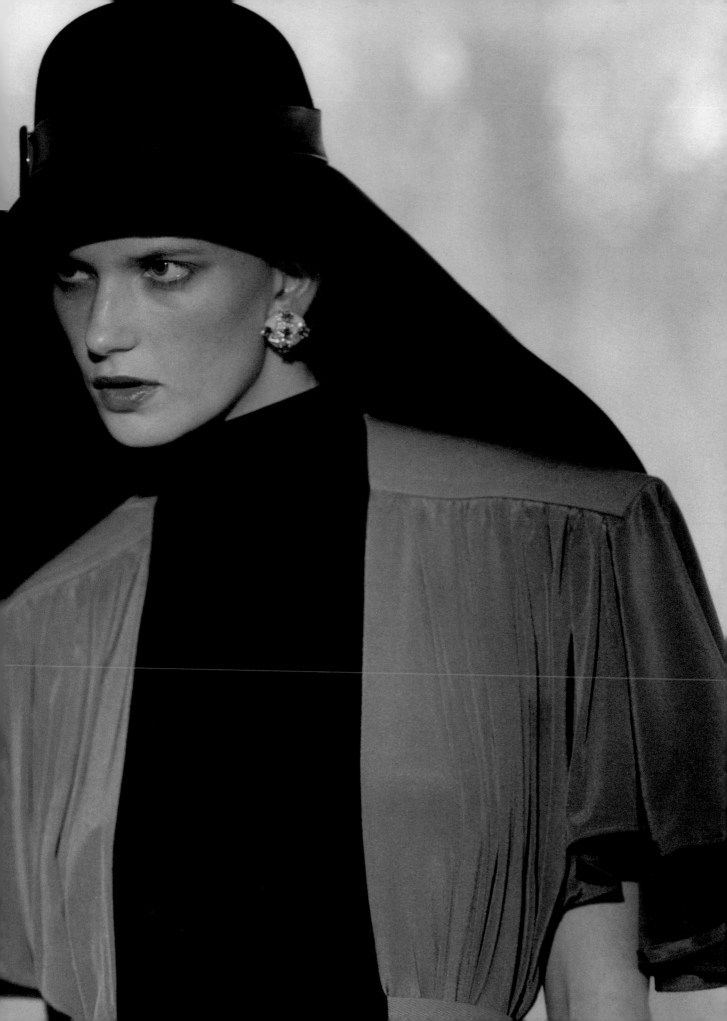

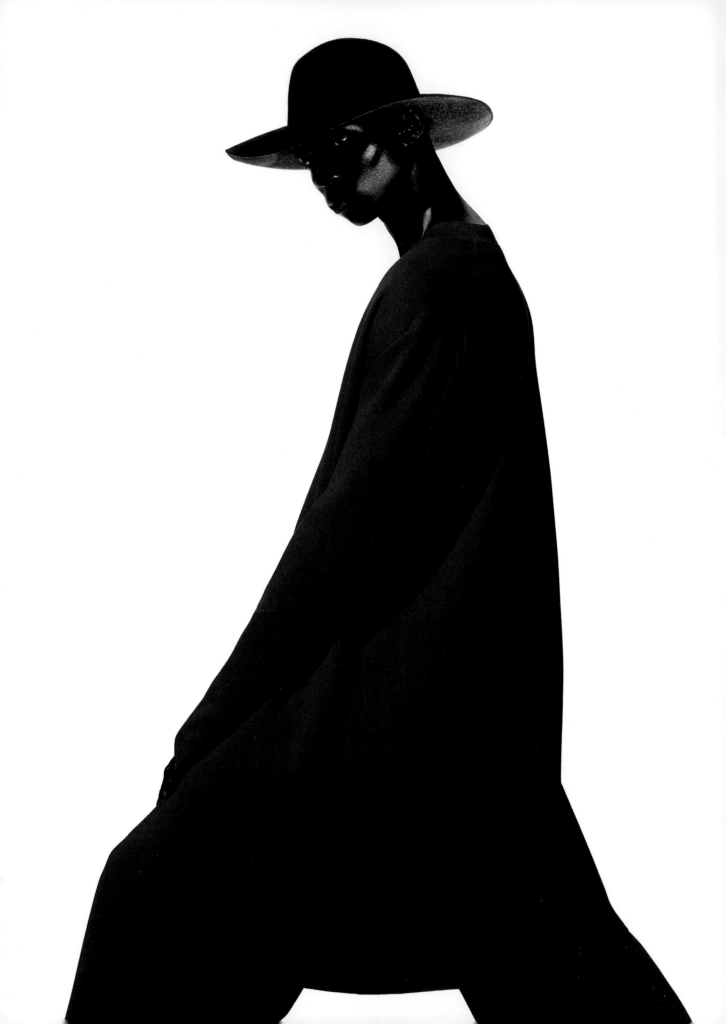

Daniel Sannwald's practice is both hi-tech and lo-fi, oscillating between digital and analogue formats.

Daniel Sannwald

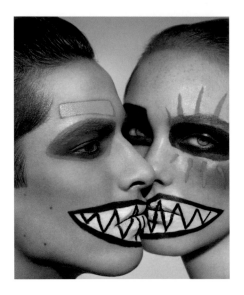

London-based, German photographer Daniel Sannwald (b. 1979) is one of the most widely published new generation fashion image-makers featured in this book. While he was still a photography student at the Royal Academy of Fine Arts in Antwerp. Sannwald's photographs were picked up by stylist Nicola Formichetti, marking the beginning of an important relationship with *Dazed & Confused* and the start of his career as a professional photographer. Since then his work has appeared in magazines such as *i-D*, *032c*, *Arena Homme +*, *Pop*, *Wallpaper**, *Rebel*, *The Room*, *Qvest* and *10 Men*. His monograph, *Pluto & Charon*, was released by Ludion in 2010.

In one sense, Sannwald's unpredictable photographs, which are often loaded with indecipherable or dreamlike symbols and juxtapositions, escape literal reading or conventional description. His work is not easy: there is no consistent pattern to the look of his images, nor is there any sense of regularity in his approach to the medium, making it almost impossible to safely decode his photographs. And yet all of his pictures revel in fashion, beauty and sophisticated styling. With each new commission, he finds a radical way to represent the high-fashion garments on show.

As more and more practitioners embrace hybridity, using a range of different methods to build up eclectic portfolios of fashion work, the traditional genre or process-based interpretation of fashion imagery is becoming increasingly outmoded. Sannwald's practice is both hi-tech and lo-fi, oscillating between digital and analogue formats, and mixing up what might once have been thought of as portrait, still-life and conceptual frameworks, although none of these genres can adequately define what he does. Early photographs featured in *Pluto & Charon*, such as the double-portrait cover for *Dazed & Confused* from 2008, were shot on film. That same year he made his first computer-generated images with set designer Gary Card for a Louis Vuitton story published in *Vogue Hommes Japan*. From flip phones to thermal cameras, Sannwald embraces many different technologies, sometimes as an experiment, but often simply because the equipment is close to hand. Rather than attempting to master the latest digital techniques, however, he draws our attention to the artifice of the promise of the new.

Sannwald's photographs are visually complex and rarely straightforward. He frequently builds up areas of digital effect, creating additional layers of visual information over the surface of his subjects' bodies. His models' skin often appears to have been stripped away, producing an effect that recalls the moment in a science-fiction narrative when the anthropomorphic outer shell of an android is ruptured to reveal the deception beneath: a melancholic tangle of wires and circuit boards rather than human flesh and blood. Sometimes the layers of effect are more seamless – the 'skins' shiny and intact, and perhaps a little too perfect – while at other times it is as though a blip or bug has disrupted an image on a computer monitor. In Sannwald's most extreme photographs (so far), figures are broken down completely into pixelated colour blocks.

Although we might think of Sannwald as a studio photographer, his studio exists primarily on a virtual level, rather than being the traditional, physical working space that has played such an important part in the history of fashion photography. Consequently, the 'sets' we see on the printed page are often abstract or fantastical digital constructions, rarely alluding to any sense of 'real' place.

200 'Untitled', *Arena Homme +*, 2011 — **202** 'Untitled', *Dazed & Confused*, 2008 — **202** 'Untitled', *Arena Homme +*, 2012
204 'Untitled', *Pop*, 2012 — **205 above** 'Untitled', *Arena Homme +*, 2012 — **205 below** 'Untitled', *Interview*, 2012
206–207 'Untitled', *Vogue Hommes Japan*, 2008

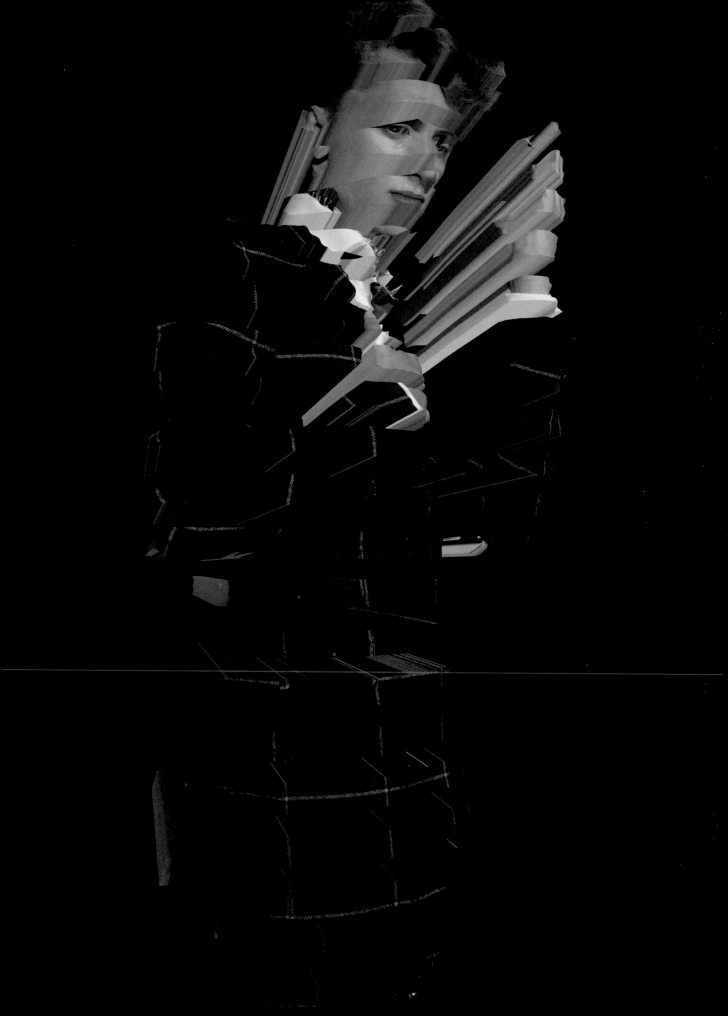

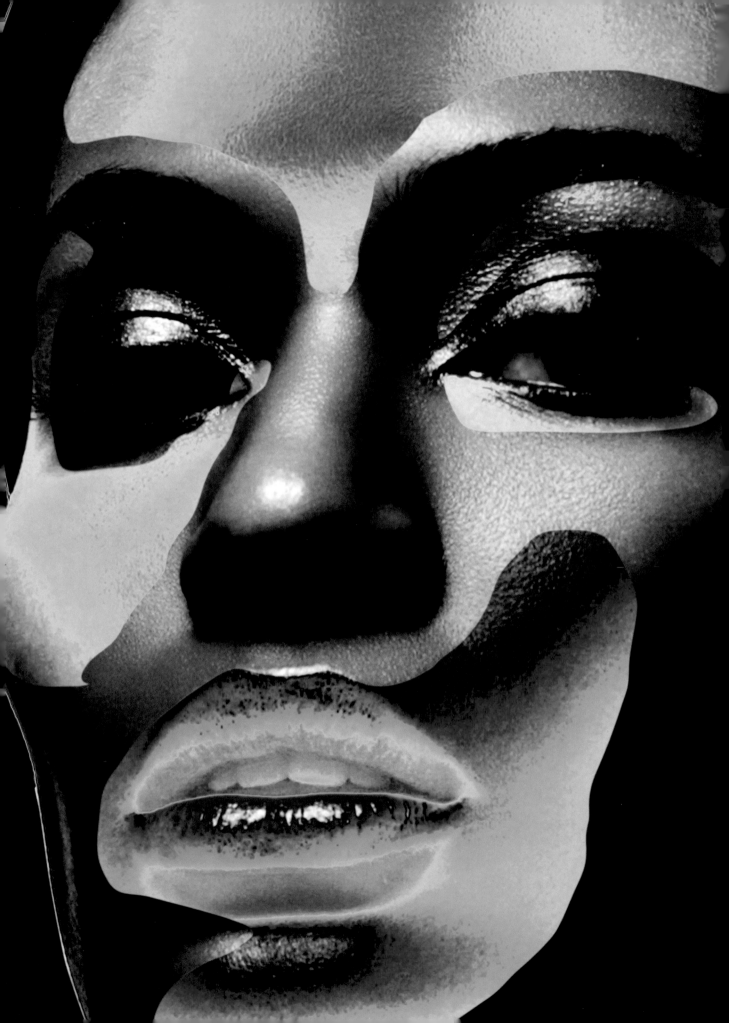

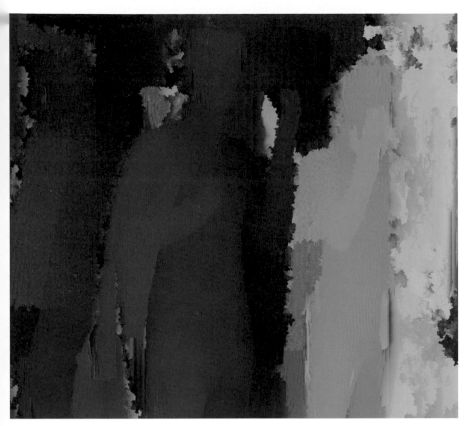

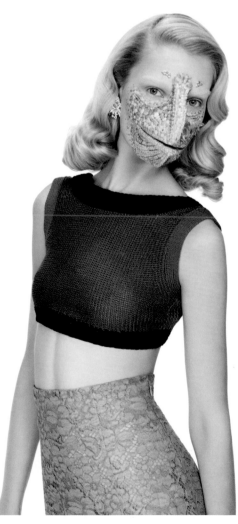

Daniel Sannwald

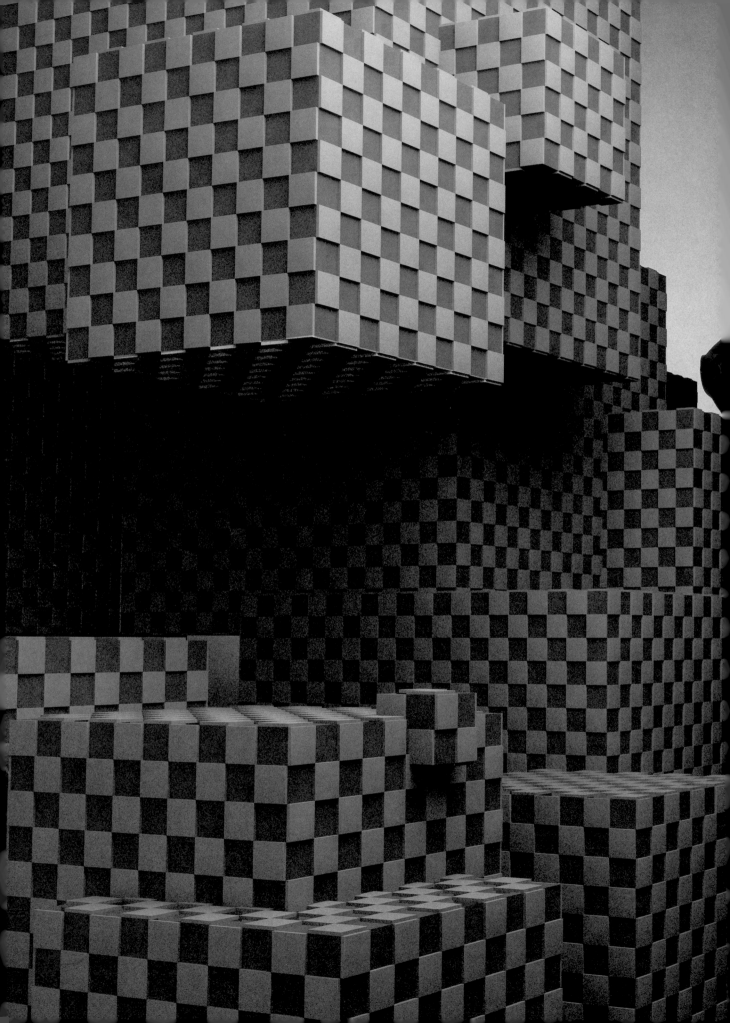

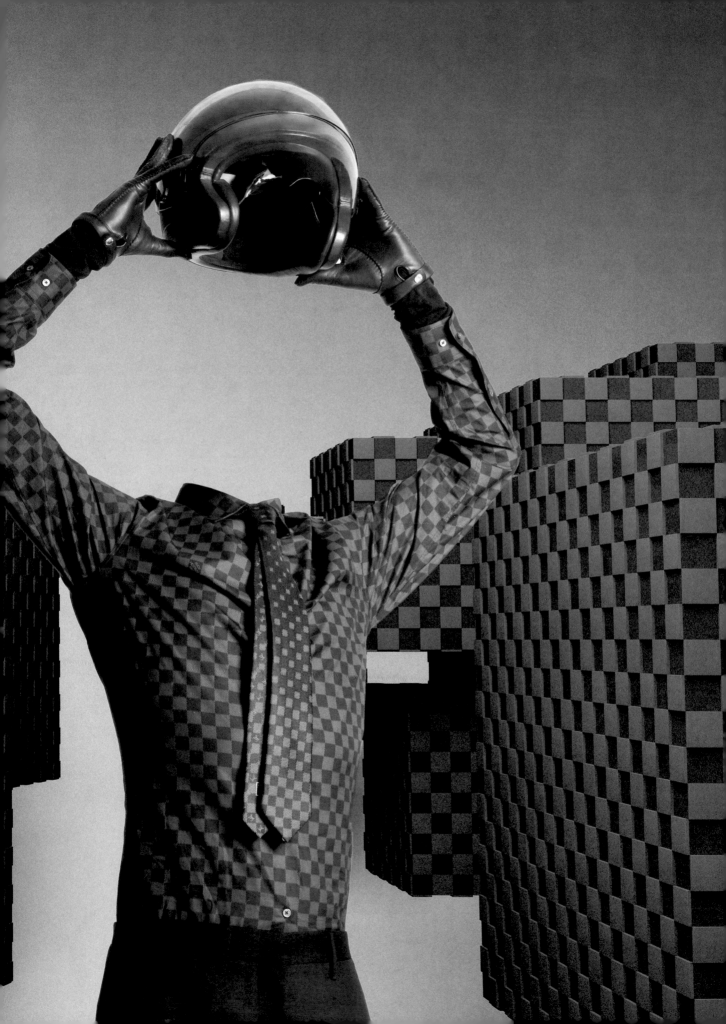

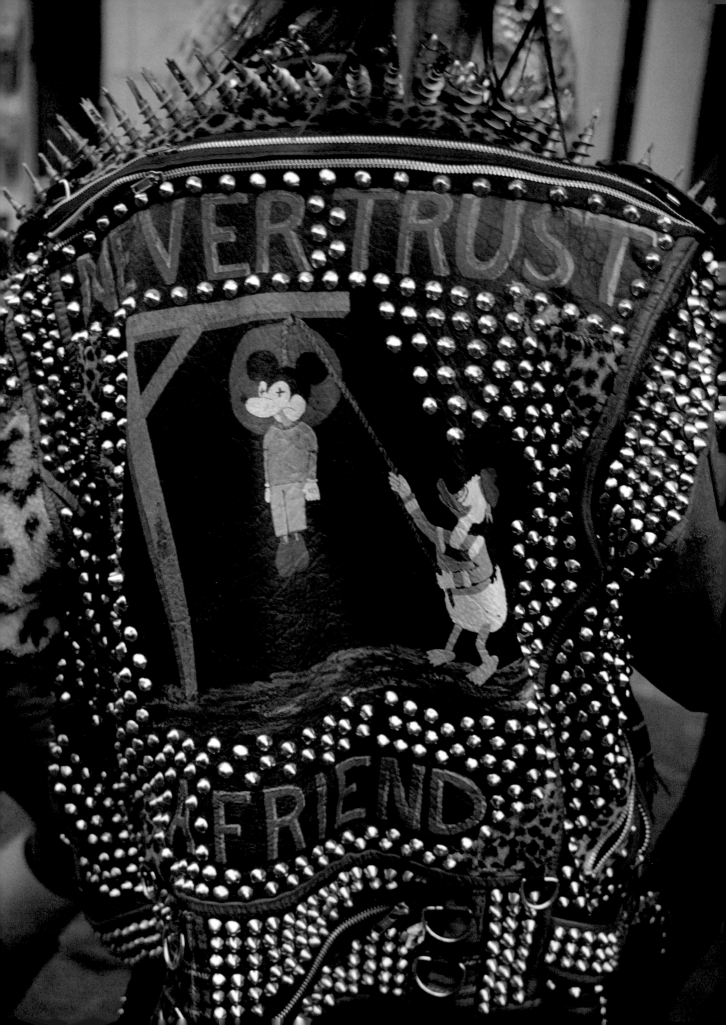

Dennis Schoenberg explores fashion as part of the creation of identity, desire and belonging.

Dennis Schoenberg

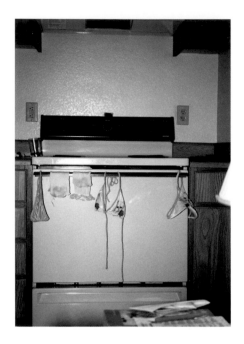

Dennis Schoenberg (b. 1978) was born in West Berlin. He moved to London in 1995 and has been based there ever since, apart from a brief stint working as a photographer's assistant in New York. He holds a BA in film and audio-visual production, as well as an MA in photography from the University of Westminster. Before starting out on his own, Schoenberg assisted Rankin, Steven Klein and Wolfgang Tillmans. Each of these experiences informed his work in a different way, and he gained incredible insight into portrait, fashion and fine-art photography respectively.

Schoenberg's break came in 2003 when Terry Jones offered him the chance to shoot editorials for *i-D* magazine. He continues to produce features for *i-D* on a regular basis, as well as working on commissions for publications such as *Vogue*, *Qvest*, *Hero*, *Exit*, *Art Review*, *Sang Bleu*, *Clash*, *Die Zeit*, *The Observer*, *SHOWstudio*, and many more. Besides his fashion work, Schoenberg has shot portraits of actors Marion Cotillard and Mark Ruffalo, singer-songwriters Patti Smith and Pete Doherty, filmmaker Wong Kar-Wai, stylist Edward Enninful, writer Bret Easton Ellis and designer Katharine Hamnett, among others.

A very early proponent of digital technology, Schoenberg does occasionally use film, but continues to work mostly with digital cameras. Inspired by art, music and cinema, as well as by the people around him, he often embarks on personal projects as a way to understand a particular region or place, or in an attempt to translate into image a philosophical concept he sees evidenced in social phenomena. For example, his series *Politics*, which documents the run-down facades of amusement arcades in Blackpool, northern England, points to the French philosopher Paul Valéry's definition of politics as 'the art of preventing people from taking part in affairs which properly concern them'.

Schoenberg's practice tends to blur the lines between what is and what is not traditionally defined as fashion imagery. This is seen clearly in his ongoing fascination with and documentation of punk subculture in the UK. His subjects' unconventional, deconstructive and often anarchic approach to fashion is a hugely important part of his reportage-style photographs. The implication here is that fashion photography is not simply about about stylish, high-end design and on-trend labels; it is also about the creation of identity, desire and belonging, and the capturing of a precise moment or story. Even if an image claims to have no interest in fashion, the garments, accessories and hairstyles on display can evoke a certain mood.

As we can see, Schoenberg has a much broader understanding of fashion photography than many of his contemporaries, using his camera to question what makes people shape their external appearance and way of life around a particular look. An awareness of this expanded notion of the role of fashion in society is key to our interpretation of his work. For Schoenberg, clothes are very much secondary in the attempt to create singular 'moments', for which not everything can be planned. His 'less is more' approach acknowledges that all his subjects are different, while simultaneously making sure that his photographs work as part of a sequence, as well as in their own right as individual portraits of a particular person, place and time.

208 'Never Trust a Friend', 2006 — **210** 'Underwear', 2000 — **211** 'Duct Leather', 2012 — **212** 'Diner', 2006
213 above 'Dean', 2007 — **213 below** 'Chris', 2007

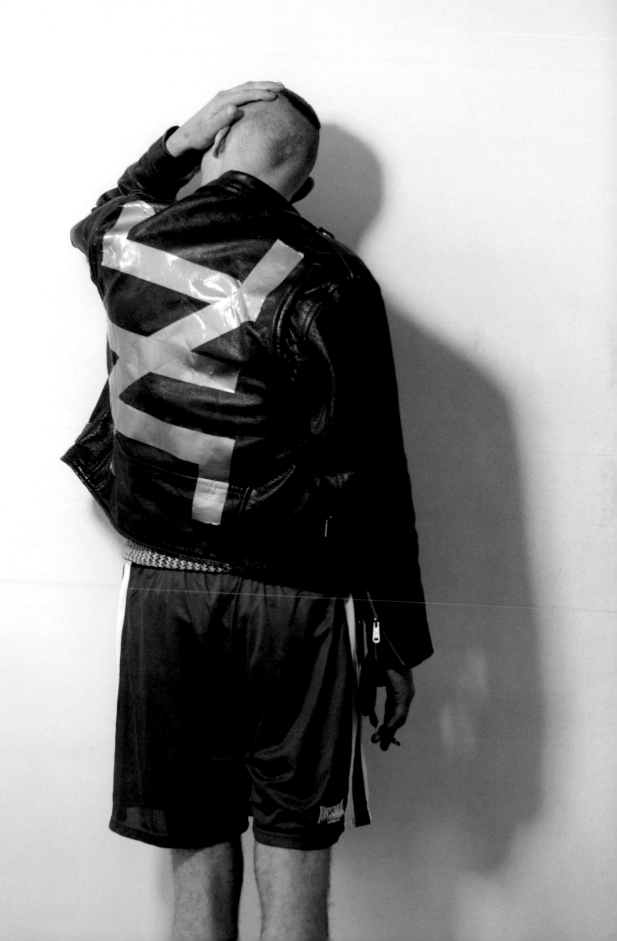

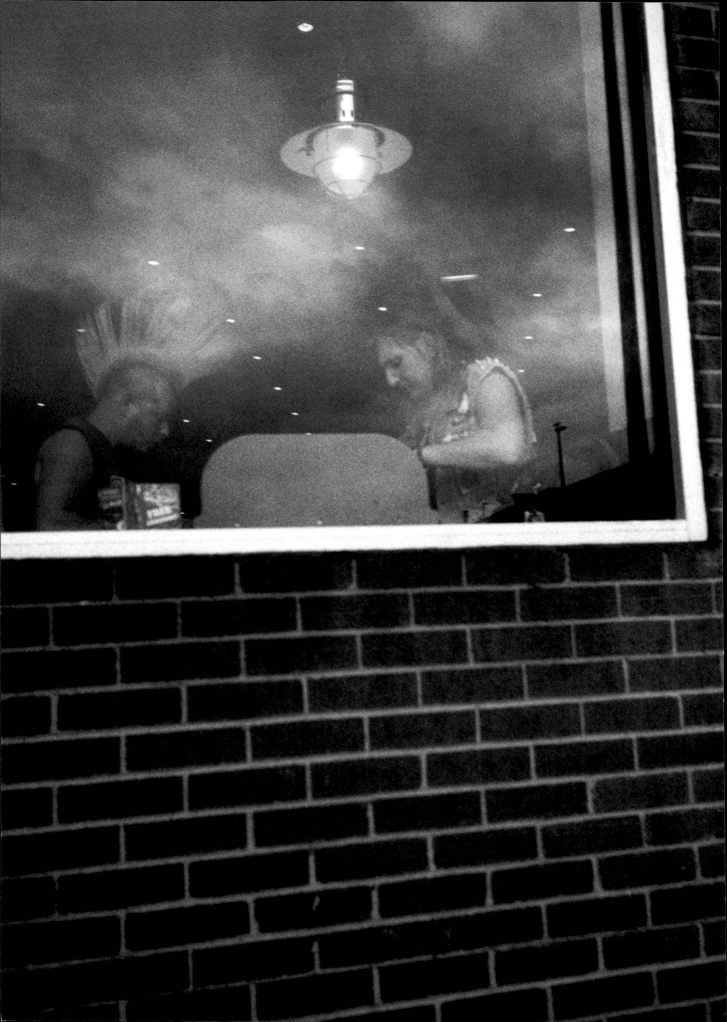

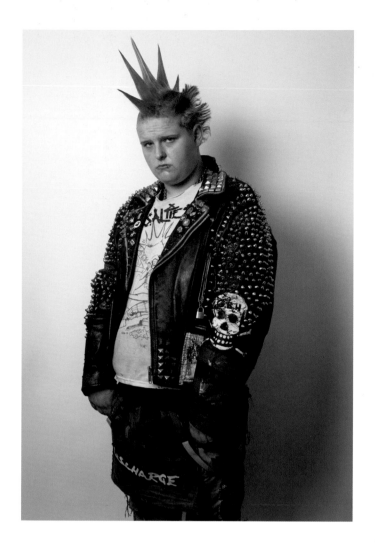

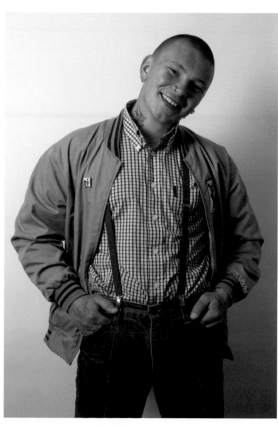

Dennis Schoenberg

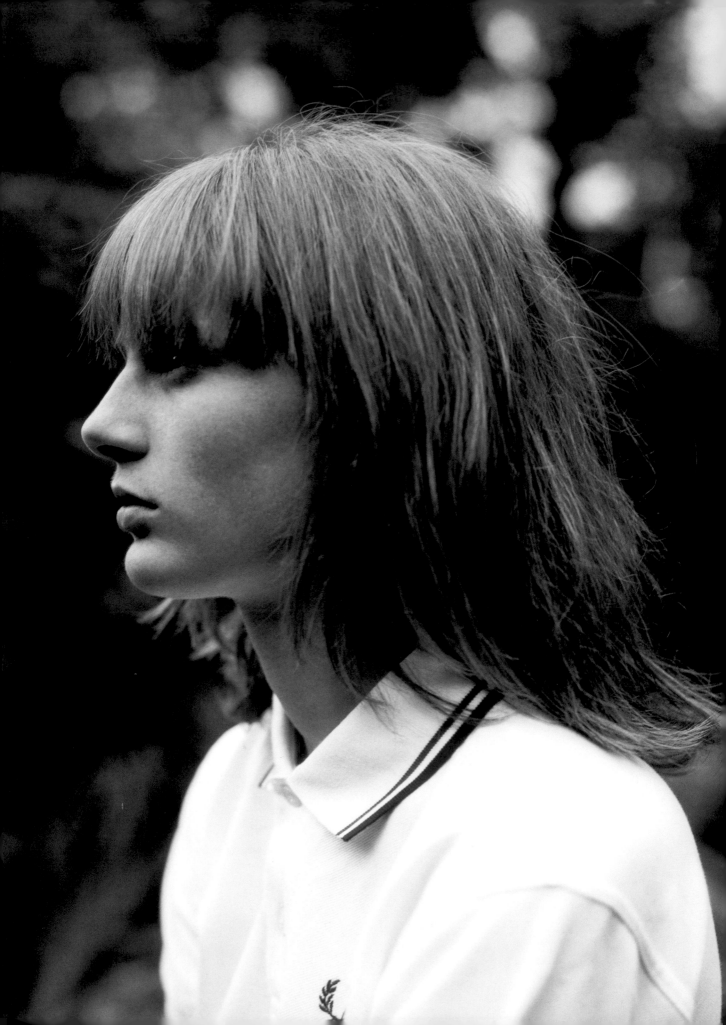

Clare Shilland tries to catch her subjects off-guard and capture in-between moments.

Clare Shilland

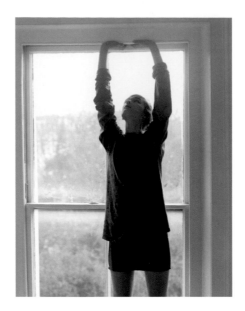

Clare Shilland (b. 1973) studied graphic design at Camberwell College of Arts before embarking on an MA in photography at the Royal College of Art, both in London. Like many photographers of her generation, she was inspired by work published in *i-D* and *The Face* during the 1990s by photographers such as Juergen Teller, Glen Luchford, Bruce Weber, Elaine Constantine and Wolfgang Tillmans. After a brief period assisting, Shilland produced her first editorial for the April 2001 issue of *Nova* magazine, and subsequently began working together with the stylist, editor and designer David Bradshaw. An early collaboration with Bradshaw for *10 Men*'s autumn/winter 2003 issue, for which she photographed female models in men's clothing, featured many of the defining traits of her work.

Shilland tends to shoot on location with subtle, gentle light – often daylight – and works with film as much as possible, using minimal post-production. She has a naturalistic, subject-led and highly personal approach towards image-making,

seeking out models with a quiet beauty for her portraits or fashion sequences. Shilland prefers not to be directorial when shooting and instead attempts to catch her subjects off-guard or capture in-between moments. In her images, fashion is often positioned as part of ordinary life. Though her photographs are staged, they propose an alternative to the extreme artifice and exaggerated poses usually associated with high-fashion imagery, a stylistic tendency with roots in work made by Norman Parkinson in the 1950s or by David Bailey in the '60s that has become more prevalent in British fashion photography since the end of the twentieth century.

More recently, Shilland has worked with stylist Michele Rafferty for Italian fashion house Marni. Rafferty commissioned Shilland and art director Dean Langley to make a limited-edition photobook on the label's autumn/winter 2013 menswear collections. In the book, grids or filmic strips of densely reproduced and repeated Polaroids are displayed alongside singular film images. Perhaps unusually for the brand, Shilland utilized the unconventional beauty of British

model Reece Sanders, demonstrating the continued importance of casting to her work. She skilfully elicited slight variations of pose and expression from Sanders, and the resulting stills convey a sense of spontaneity and dynamic progression.

Shilland also worked with Langley on shoots for *Beat*, an innovative music magazine founded by Hanna Hanra in 2010 and distributed for free around London. Other collaborative projects include her ongoing *Love From...* series of independent publications with stylist Beth Fenton and graphic designers Wood McGrath. The first book, a collection of photographs taken in London in 2008, was a beguiling abstract fictional narrative developed around the idea of the postcard.

In 2010, Shilland was the winner of the *Elle* Commission at the Taylor Wessing Photographic Portrait Prize, sponsored by the National Portrait Gallery in London. The following year, her work was included as part of the DoBeDo collective in the exhibition 'The Arsenal: 125' at the Saatchi Gallery, also in London.

214 'Louise Profile', *10 Men*, 2003 — 216 'Lara Window', *i-D*, 2013 — 217 'Alice' from *Love from Alice*, 2010
218 'Melissa', *The Gentlewoman*, 2010 — 219 Reece Sanders, *Marni Uomo*, A/W 2013

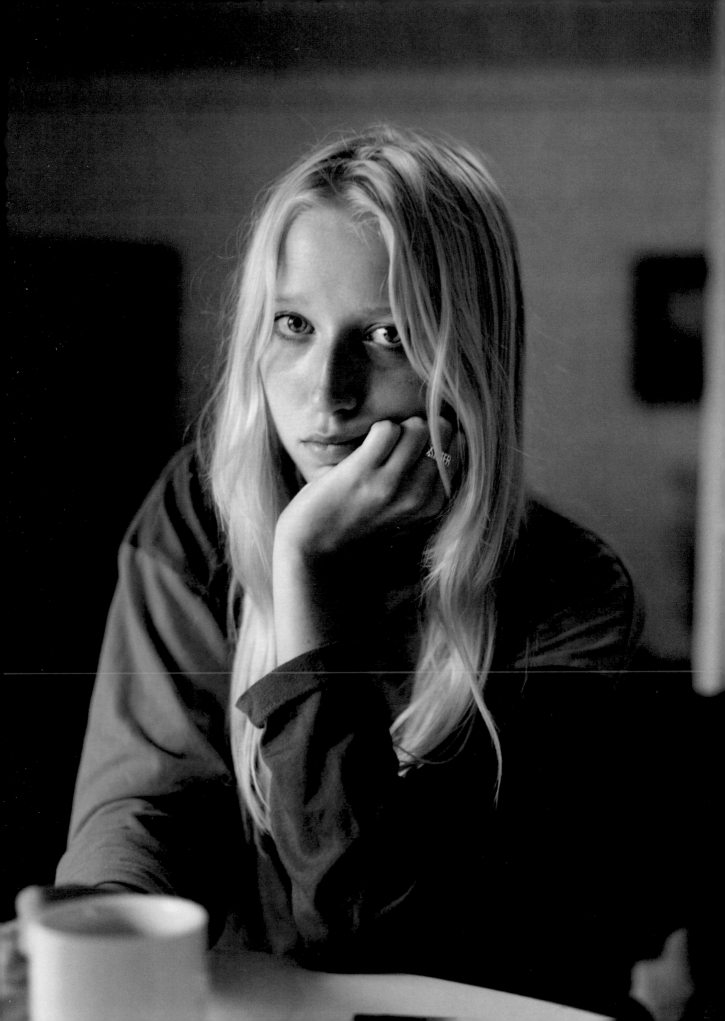

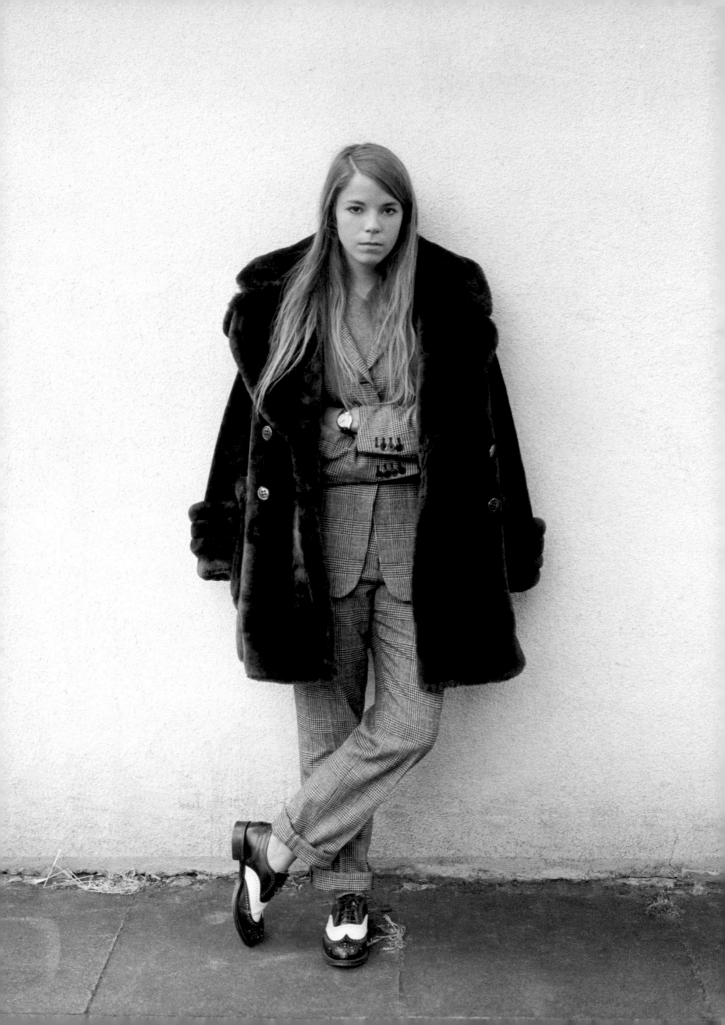

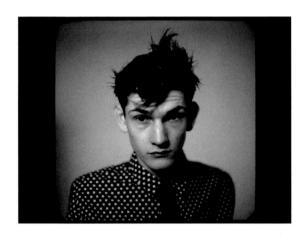
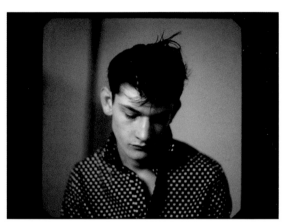
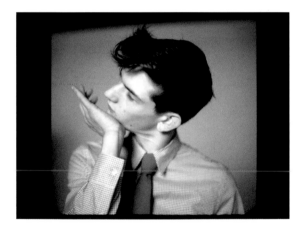
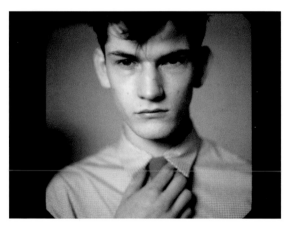

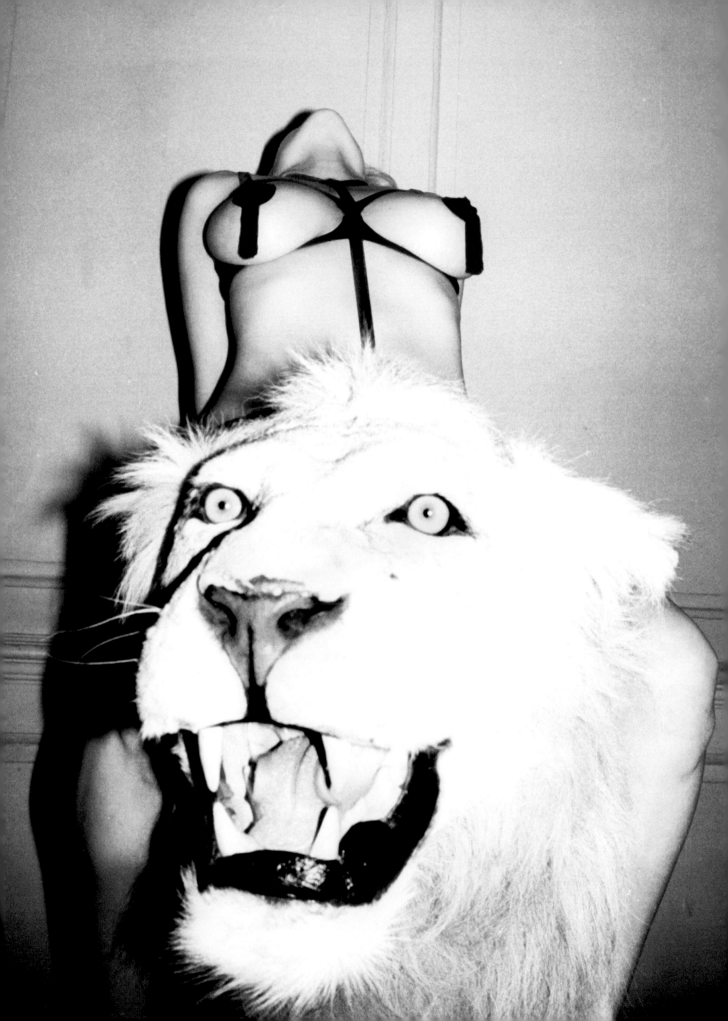

Saga Sig's interests centre on the fantastical and her desire to create alternative worlds.

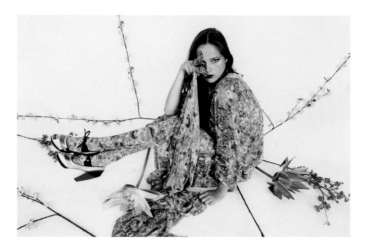

Saga Sigurðardottir (b. 1986), better known as Saga Sig, is an Icelandic photographer based in London. She grew up in Þingvellir National Park, south-west Iceland, where she was inspired at an early age by the way the light transforms the landscape throughout the seasons. Wanting to capture the dramatic beauty of Icelandic nature, Sig started taking photographs when she was 8 years old after receiving her first camera from her parents. Some years later, during her first year at the University of Iceland in Reykjavik, where she was enrolled on the art history course, she became the photography director of the university paper. This experience showed her how much she loved planning shoots and working with different people.

Although she had always been inspired by light, colour, form and texture, with a strong desire to tell stories, Sig never intended to become a professional photographer and was not particularly interested in fashion until she was about 19, when she started working in a vintage store. She subsequently became engrossed in patterns, fabrics and finishings, and began organizing small shoots with the clothes.

Fashion photography eventually became an obvious career choice for Sig. In September 2009, after finishing her first year at the University of Iceland, she moved to the UK to study fashion photography at the London College of Fashion, where she met many of the people with whom she continues to collaborate today. While there, she realized her further compatibility with fashion image-making as it facilitates (and arguably necessitates) teamwork. Many disparate elements need to come together to create a beautiful image that can tell a story, so it is incredibly important for a photographer to have an 'amazing team'.

Sig's photographs have appeared in British, Japanese and Korean *Dazed & Confused*, Mexican and Japanese *Nylon*, and on *i-D*'s website. Since graduating from the London College of Fashion in 2011, she has continued to shoot editorials and other commercial fashion features while simultaneously pursuing the personal interests that form the core of her practice and were the reason for her choosing photography in the first place. These interests centre on the fantastical and her desire to create alternative worlds and different characters. She predominantly

uses film, preferring to shoot on location with natural light. Sig has also maintained her enthusiasm for photographing nature, and more recently has experimented with still-life photography, often building her own mini sets.

Every day is different for Sig: she relishes in the fact that her profession continually enables her to meet new people, see new places and explore a range of human emotions. There is an unmistakable sense of mysticism to her photographs. Although some of her images are sexualized, her distinct gaze as a woman prevents them from becoming salacious; instead, the pictures celebrate the natural beauty that can be found equally in the Icelandic landscape, the curve of a woman's breast, or the artful assemblage of colour and line in a gown. With this in mind, it is no surprise that when asked which photographers she most admires, Sig mentions Nobuyoshi Araki. Although the Japanese photographer gained notoriety for his erotic images of bound women, it is his lesser known personal work – his street photography and intimate studies of his wife – that Sig appreciates. She describes his work as 'so human; about death, love and sex'.

————

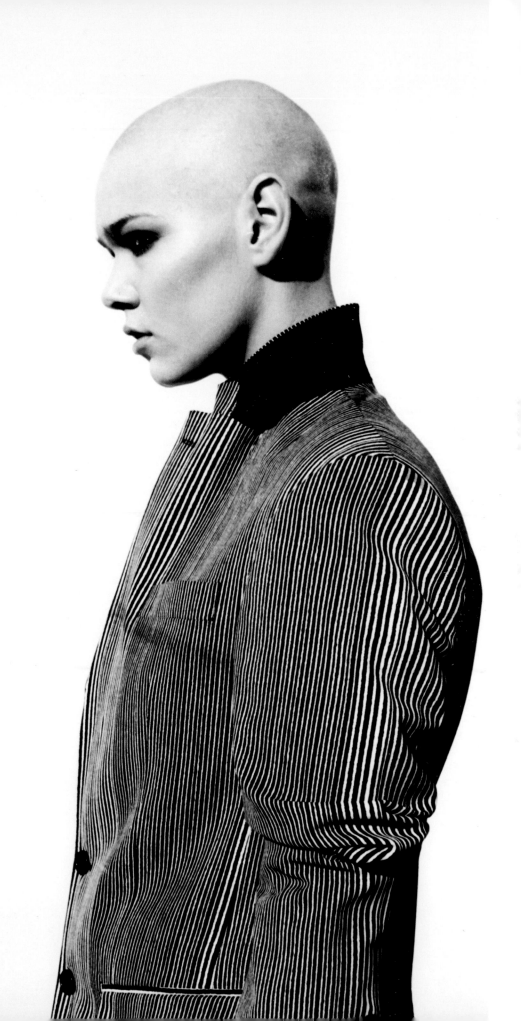

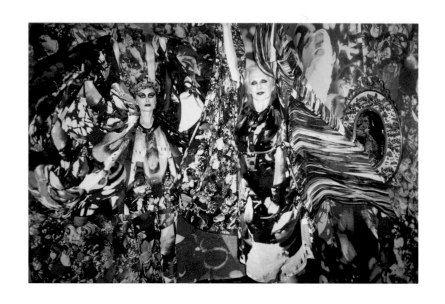

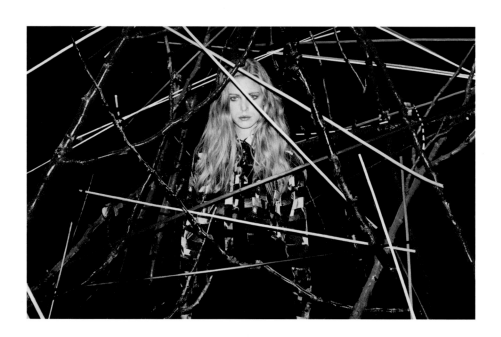

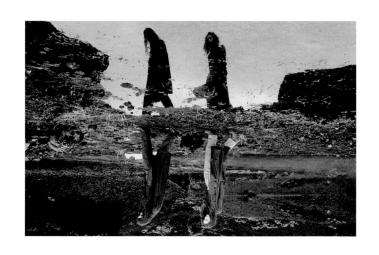

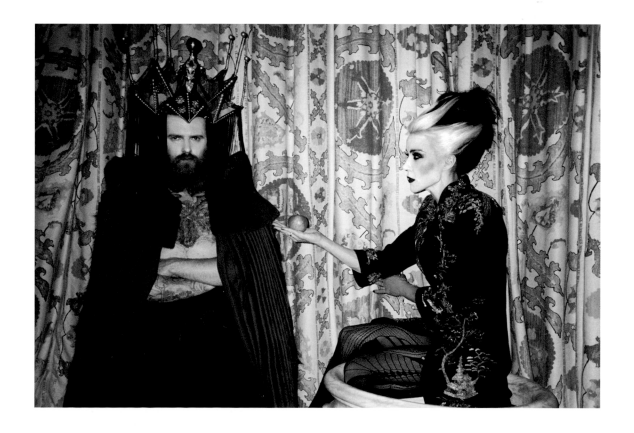

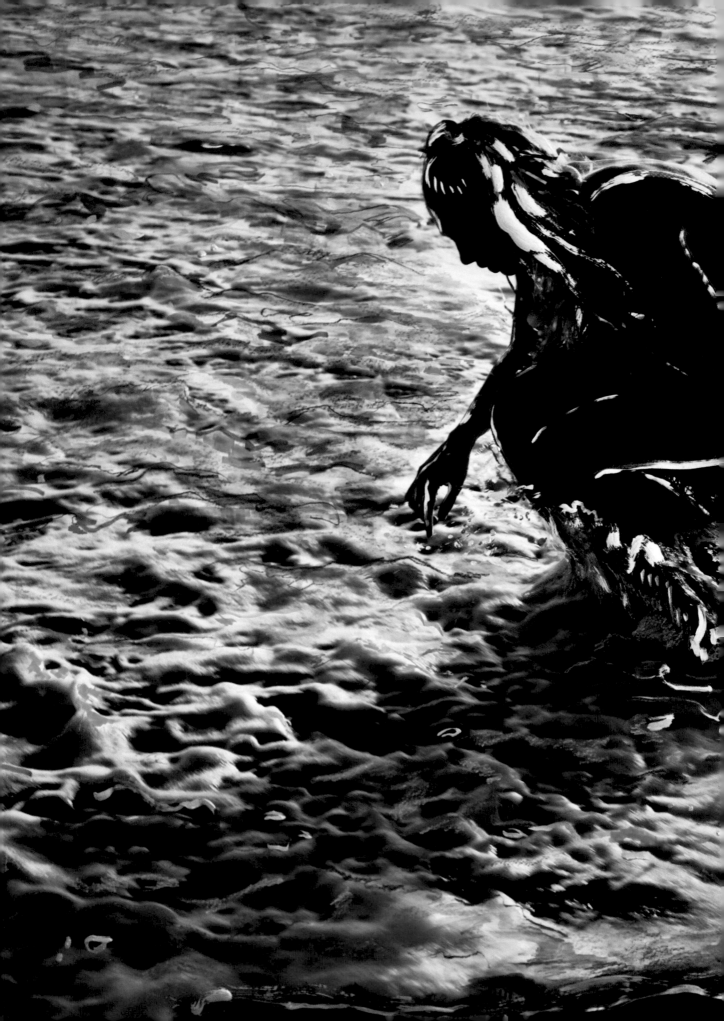

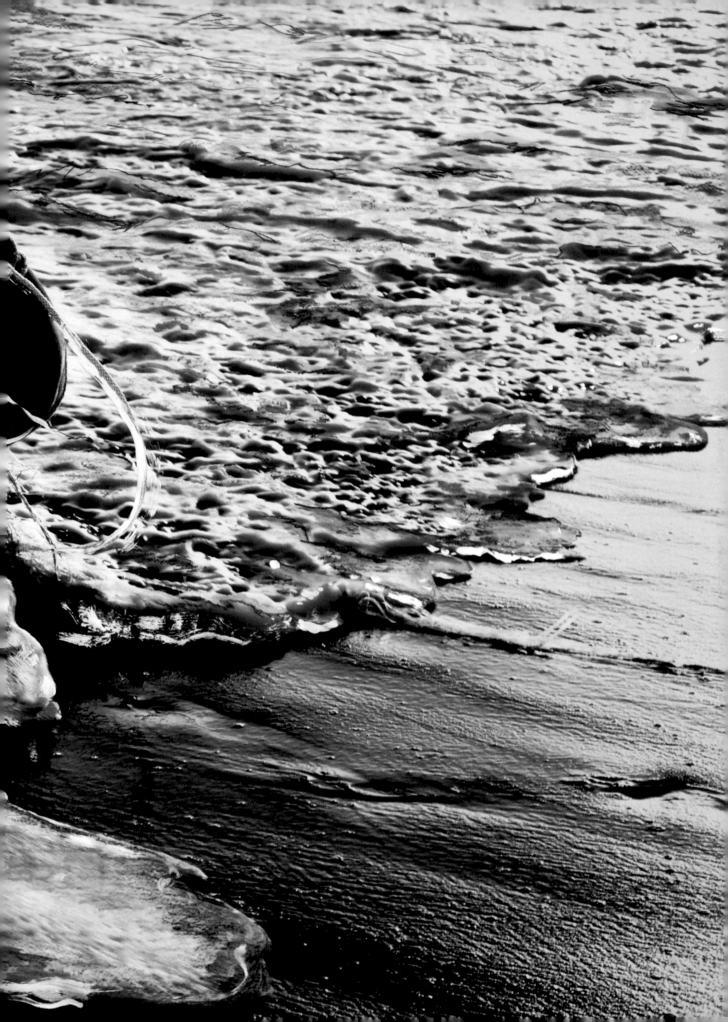

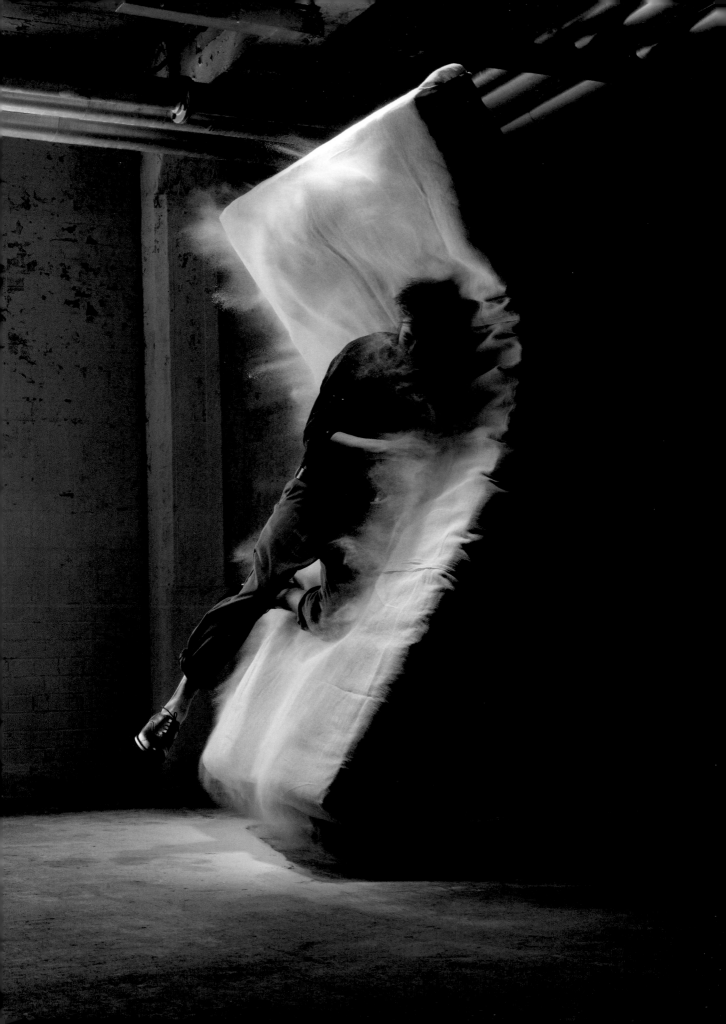

Jacob Sutton's work is less narrative and more experiential than that of many of his contemporaries.

Jacob Sutton

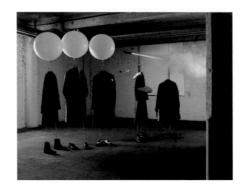

Jacob Sutton (b. 1979) is set to make a significant contribution to British fashion photography, continuing the intensely rich period of creativity that began in the UK in the 1990s. Originally from Bath, he moved to London in 1999 to study photography at the London College of Printing (now London College of Communication). After several years spent assisting, during which time he worked with British photographers Dan Tobin Smith, Liz Collins and John Akehurst, Sutton produced his first fashion story for *Dazed & Confused* in 2005. His early editorials garnered considerable industry recognition, marking him out as part of the new wave of exceptional talent and demonstrating his potential to become one of most interesting photographers of his generation. Sutton's images have appeared in numerous magazines – from the establishment masthead *Vogue* to *i-D*, *Interview* and *AnOther/AnOther Man* – and his commercial clients include Burberry, Y-3, Hermès, Loewe, Bergdorf Goodman and Topman.

Sutton makes both studio and location-based fashion images. His best work is less narrative and more experiential than that of many of his contemporaries. In his photographs, the human body is often the physical trigger for a demonstration of concepts such as balance, cause and effect, speed, motion, gravity or impact. By making such abstract states the subject or structure of his images, Sutton has begun to progress towards an articulation of the basic elements of space and time. 'Big Bang', for example, was an editorial created for *Mixte* in 2007 with stylist Celestine Cooney, with whom Sutton frequently collaborates. Here, a comparison could be made to Swiss artists Fischli and Weiss's 1987 work *The Way Things Go*, a film about the chain reaction between objects where there is a similar sense of controlled chaos as well as an obvious enjoyment in the construction of the scene. In Sutton's story, a Dadaist collection of overcoats and shoes strung together like puppets collapse to the ground as the white balloon heads that hold them up are popped in sequence by the path of a missile. A subsequent image shows the aftermath of this domino-like fall, with the coats lying in piles on the floor.

'Look Before You Leap', a 2008 collaboration with fashion editor and stylist Elliott Smedley for *10 Men* magazine, is one of the most accomplished fashion editorials to be produced by an emerging photographer in recent years. Shot on location at a farm in the Cotswolds, the sequence of photographs brilliantly expressed the physical concepts of balance and force. In one image, a model pushes himself against a wall as a pile of precariously stacked tyres pushes back at him. In another, he sits atop a wooden cube, the last and most unstable element in a towering sculptural assemblage. Sutton used timber supports to create an angle reminiscent of American photographer Irving Penn's famous corner portraits in a sophisticated paraphrasing of one of the greatest compositional innovations ever made by a fashion photographer. A third image, in which the model's hands and feet are propped up on uneven blocks, creates a dialogue between surfaces: from the shiny black boots and buttons, and fluid cut and fall of the fabrics, to the roughness of the wooden blocks and cement bricks that support the figure. Sutton's visualization of balance complicates the notion of time, suggesting moments before and after what we see in the picture.

Sutton is well known for his work with fashion film. 'Danceteria', his video and series of photographs made with choreographer Jonah Bokaer and stylist Bruce Pask for *T: The New York Times Style Magazine* in 2009, explored the potential ambiguity between still and moving image. In the video, the models' free-flowing, intuitive, improvised movements are enhanced by the rhythmic beats of the musical score. In the stills, however, this dynamism is frozen, emphasizing intricate details of shape and gesture in such a way that the clothes worn by the dancers seem to perform. Once again, Sutton's photographs allude to a time beyond the split second captured in the frames.

228 & 230 'Powder', *Mixte*, 2007 — **231** 'Lil Buck', 2011 — **232** 'Look Before You Leap', *10 Men*, 2008
233 'Danceteria', *T: The New York Times Style Magazine*, 2009

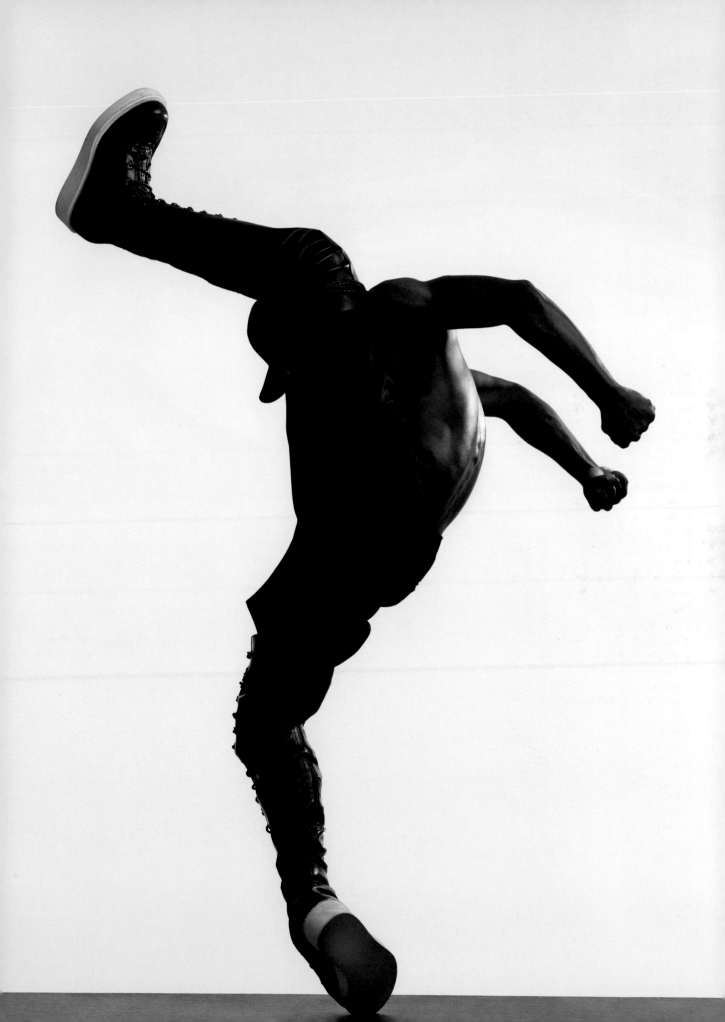

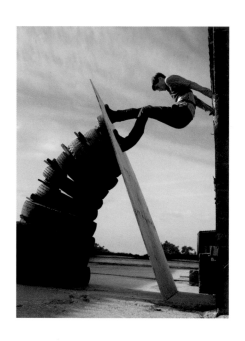

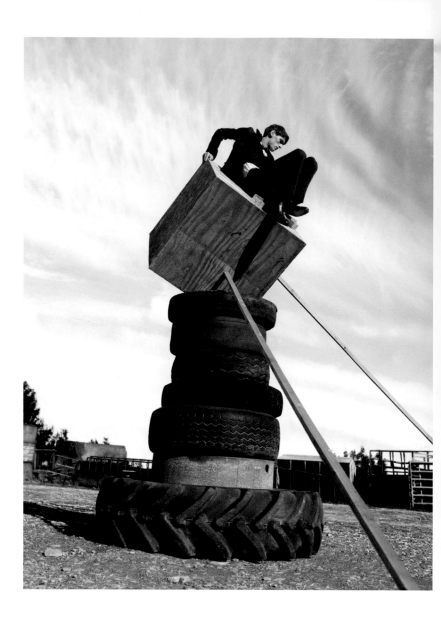

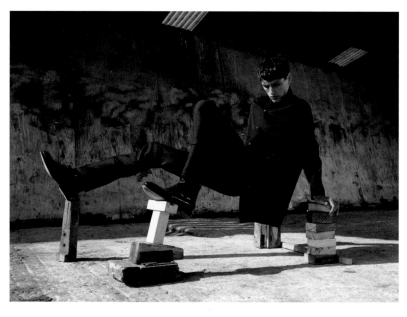

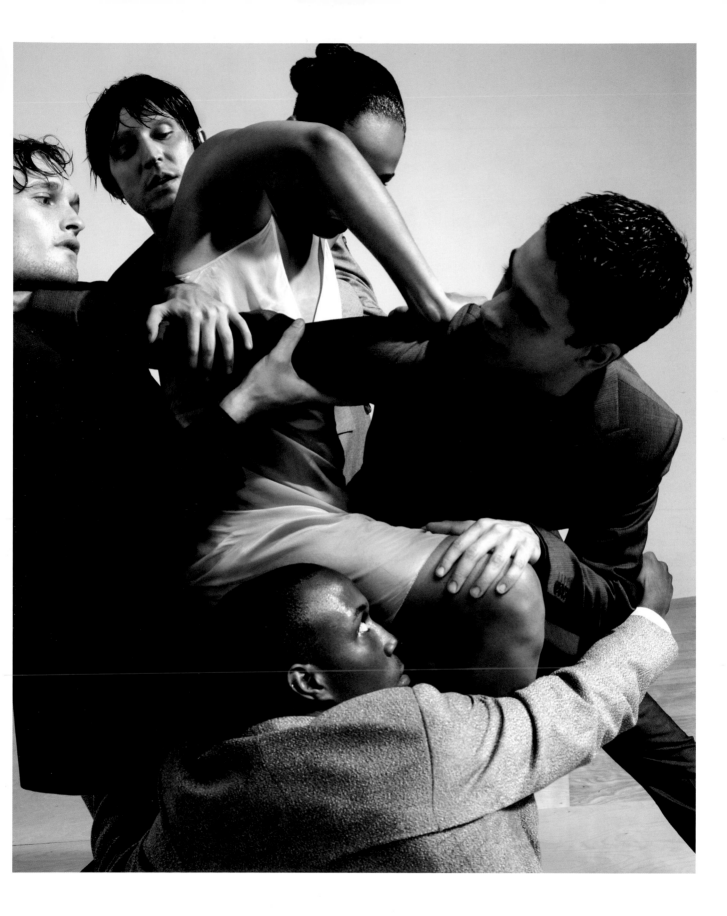

Jacob Sutton

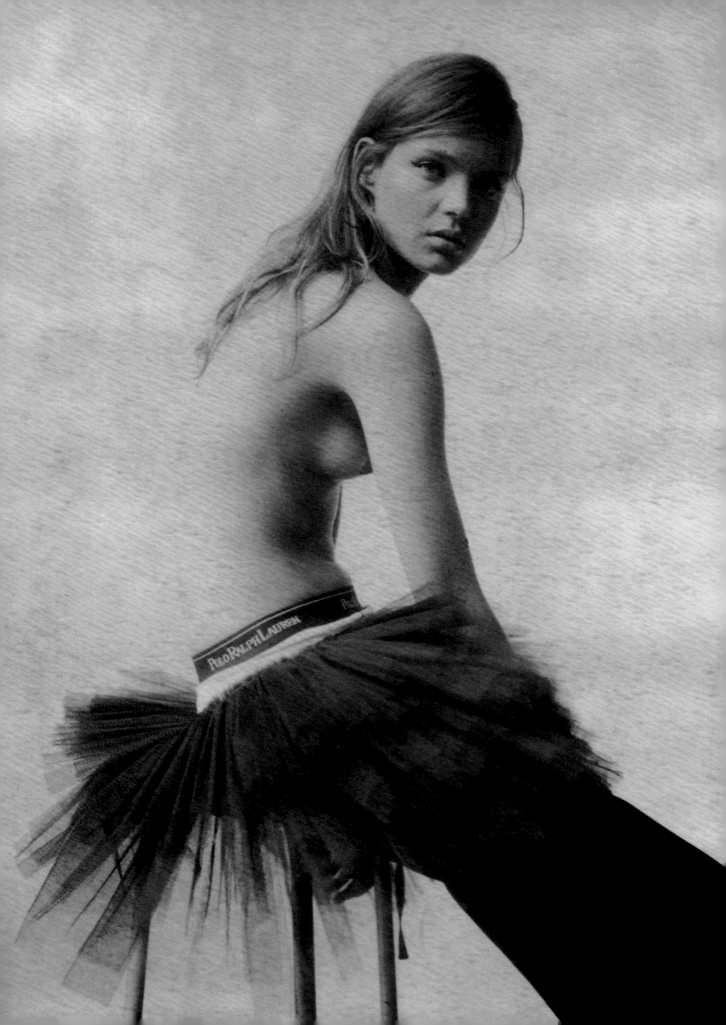

Philippe Vogelenzang aims to show people at their most powerful, confident and sincere.

Philippe Vogelenzang

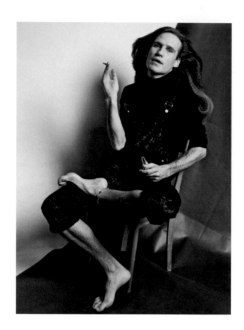

Dutch photographer Philippe Vogelenzang (b. 1982) arrived at photography in a roundabout way. After initially studying design and styling, he switched to art history for two years, before finally enrolling in the photography course he had been considering taking for a long time at the Royal Academy of Art in The Hague. After a year there, however, he decided he could learn more from practising photography than studying it. He quit his degree and started out on his own, working on model test shoots to establish a name for himself and eventually signing with an agent.

Vogelenzang's skill for making beautiful images was evident from the beginning and his career accelerated rapidly. His ongoing professional relationship with *L'Officiel Hommes NL* testifies to his consistent ability to produce strong and exciting photographs that function both independently and within fashion editorials. The Dutch magazine has allowed Vogelenzang to refine his brand of fashion imagery and develop what has now become his signature style, notably in relation to his work with men's fashion. He explains that he never made a conscious decision to principally shoot menswear, but that the opportunities to do so became more and more frequent; consequently, he has become known for his photographs of male models. A study of his images of both men and women reveals an equal attention to gesture, however, as well as a similar subversion of the stereotypical poses assigned to the different genders. Vogelenzang always tries to relay something of the person he is photographing – to show a side of their character or an aspect of their psychology – so that the story is believable. He likes to describe his work as 'fashion portraiture': each image is an attempt to capture and accurately portray the person he is photographing, be they model, celebrity or stranger.

Vogelenzang does not consider himself to be a hugely technical photographer. Instead, he takes a sensitive approach to the medium, working with both film and digital cameras, depending on the project. He has learned a lot from analogue and admires the depth that can be gained with Polaroid, but also appreciates the speed of digital and the potential for adjustment in post-production. He tends to work in black and white because it allows for greater focus on his subjects, lending the images a timeless, classic feel. In Vogelenzang's eyes, colour is a useful but not always necessary addition to a photograph. His desire to create 'modern classics' is linked to his innate understanding of portraiture; he believes that an image should feel real and as close as possible to its subject's essence.

No matter who they are, Vogelenzang aims to show people at their most powerful, confident and sincere. Besides *L'Officiel Hommes NL*, his work has been published in *El País*, Russian *GQ*, *I Love Fake*, *Zoo*, *VMan*, *V*, Dutch *Vogue* and *Vogue Hommes International*.

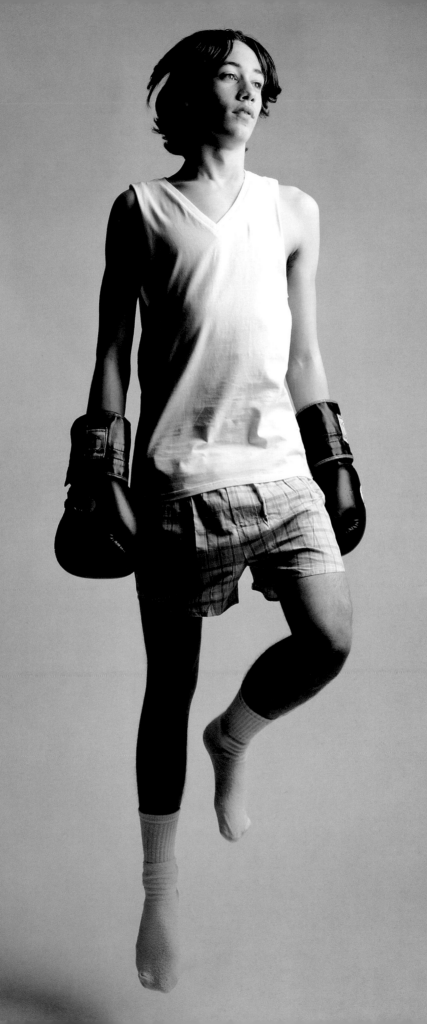

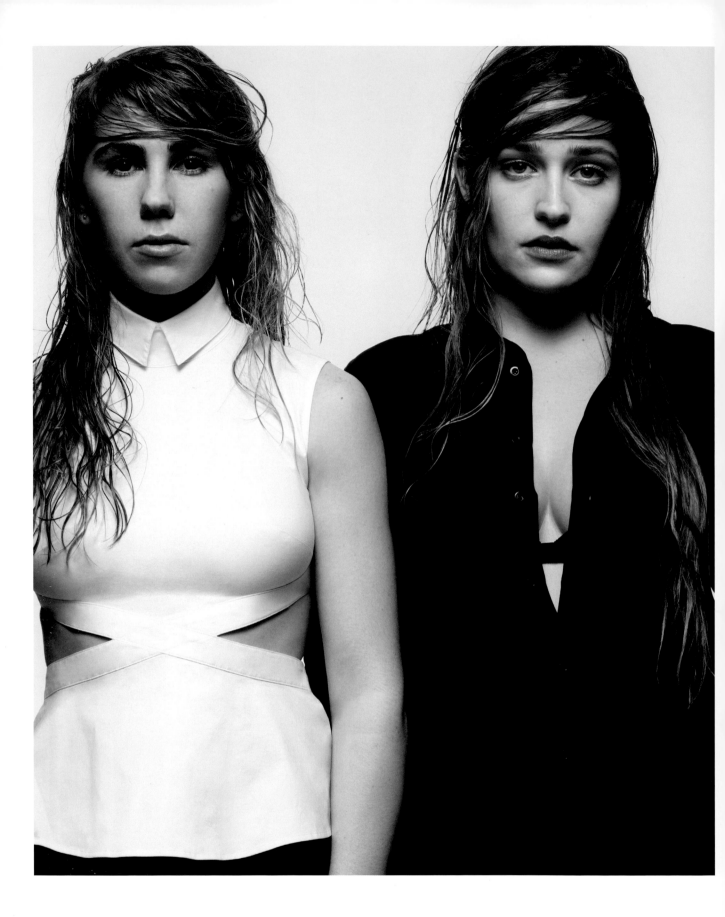

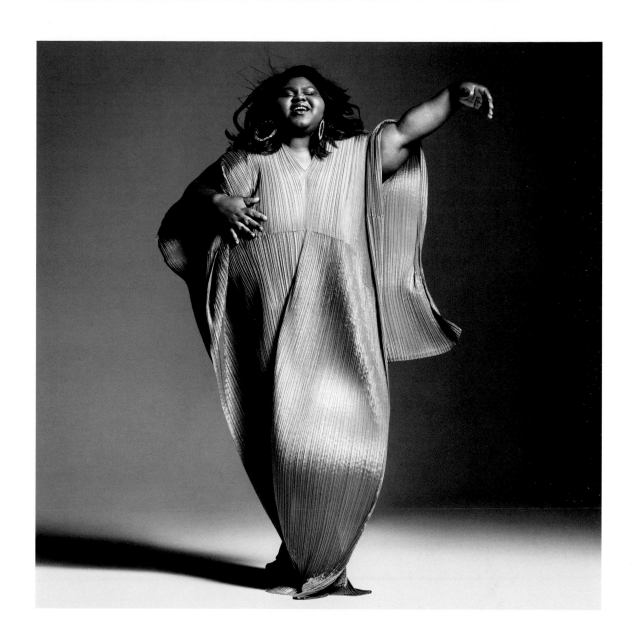

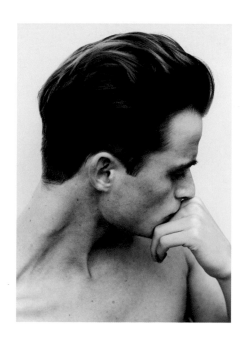

Philippe Vogelenzang

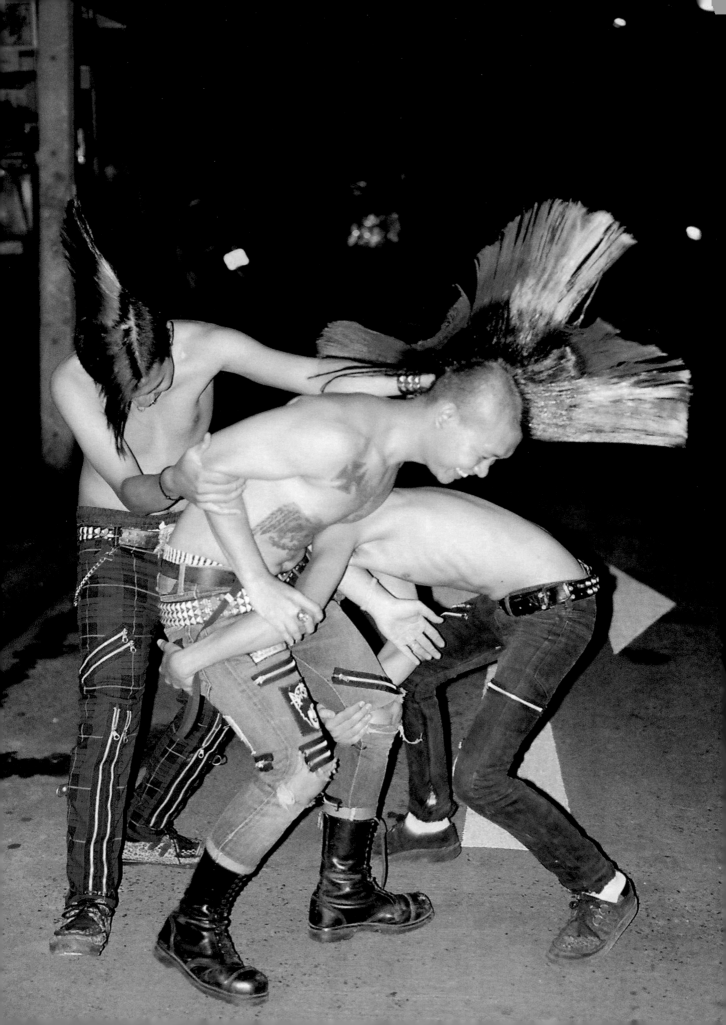

Chardchakaj Waikawee favours the snapshot for its speed and proximity to documentary photography.

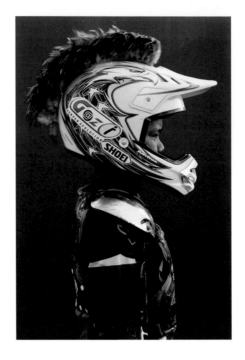

Bangkok-based, Thai photographer Chardchakaj Waikawee (b. 1980) makes fashion, portrait and documentary photographs, as well as producing television commercials and music videos. He studied at King Mongkut's Institute of Technology Ladkrabang in Bangkok, obtaining a BA in photography in 2000 and later an MA in photography and art history in 2009. He has worked at numerous Thai universities, teaching photography and related disciplines on the communication arts and design programme at Stamford International University, as well as lecturing at Bangkok University, Huachiew Chalermprakiet University and Assumption University. Besides Thailand, his work has been exhibited in Japan and the UK.

Waikawee's dynamic and varied photographic style, which prioritizes concept over rigid formal concerns, is informed by his background in moving-image production and visual communication for musicians and record labels, as well as his avid interest in sociology and psychology, particularly in relation to class. He does not consider fashion and documentary photography to be mutually exclusive – the former superficial,

the latter serious. Instead, he believes that fashion exists at the point where happiness is found in the comfort that comes from wearing clothes. With this in mind, we can understand how in his photographs fashion becomes something that can manifest itself in various ways across a range of different scenarios.

Waikawee's personal documentary-style projects reveal his interest in social issues. He has a knack for rendering social hierarchies redundant, if not absurd, through his obvious joy in his subjects and the image-making process. For example, his 2011 project *YOUTH* was a series of photographs and image installations about street teenagers in Bangkok – the young underprivileged, uneducated people abandoned by society with whom every nation can find its parallels. He captures these children and young adults in a way that evokes the careless manner in which they are treated by society, placing less emphasis on the composition of the portraits and focusing more on the moment of interaction.

The resulting images are 'unclean': blurred, out of focus, with any dust on the negative still visible on the print, they contain traces of the original encounter.

We can see something of this receptive approach to image-making in Waikawee's portrait and fashion work. He is inspired by nineteenth-century Romanticism, which influences his use of lighting and orchestration of pose, and has led him to experiment with 'every technique on every equipment and film' before eventually returning to the snapshot for its speed and proximity to documentary photography. Here, we can see the influence of his favourite photographers: Boris Mikhailov, Juergen Teller and Mark Lebon.

Waikawee's photographs are not about the equipment or technical processes he uses, but more about telling a story. He believes that his aesthetic stems from the content and intention of his images. The strength of his photographs is therefore rooted in the unique connection that exists between photographer and subject during the moment of shooting, something that can never be predetermined.

---

240 'Punk', *Playground*, 2010 — 242 'Red Rider', *MTV Trax*, 2007 — 243 'Boy' from *YOUTH*, 2012 — 244 above 'Golf', *Photo Art*, 2012
244 below 'Zmart Bikini', *DDT*, 2005 — 245 'Smoke' from *YOUTH*, 2010 — 246 'Prostitute and Her Daughter', *Photo Art*, 2012
247 above 'Boy Prostitute' from *YOUTH*, 2011 — 247 below 'BKK Gangster', *Fine Art*, 2010

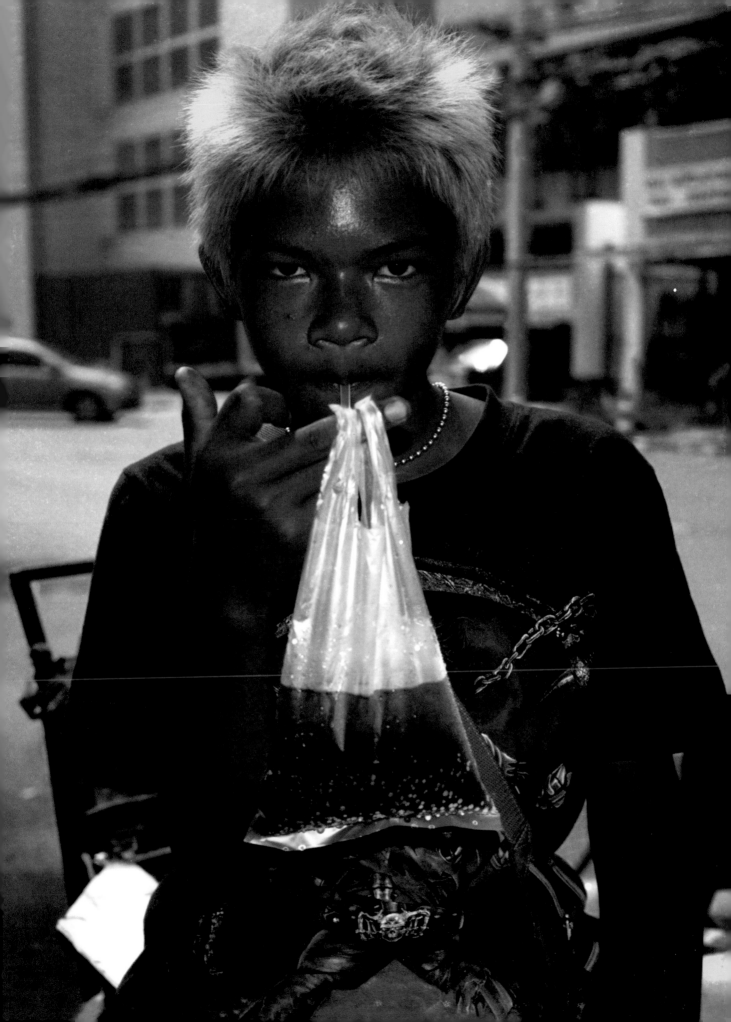

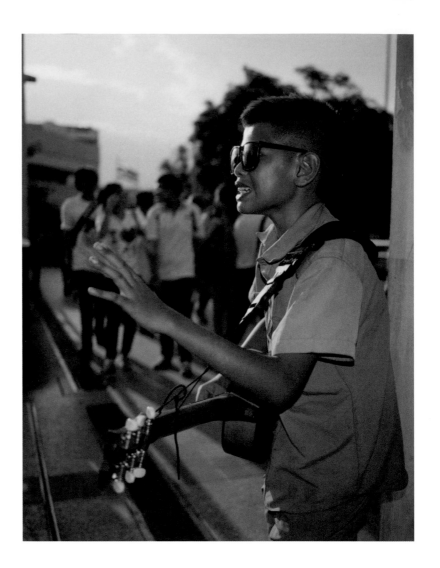

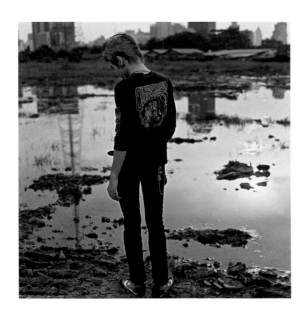

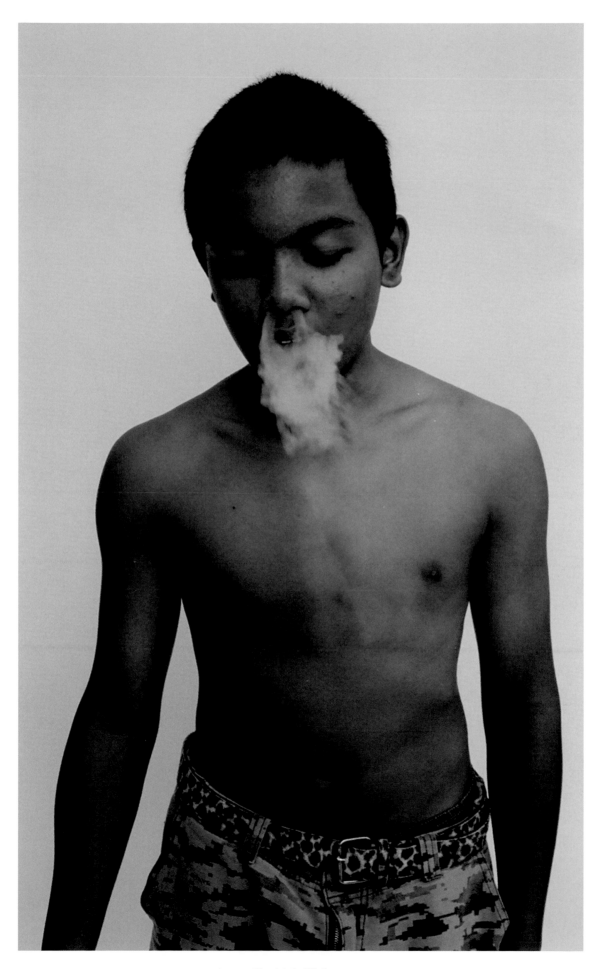

Chardchakaj Waikawee

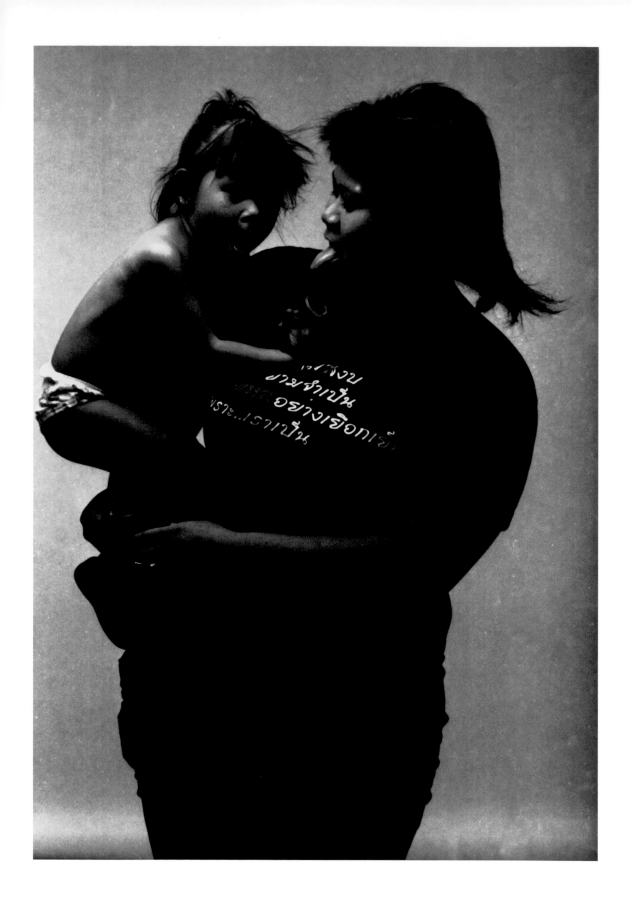

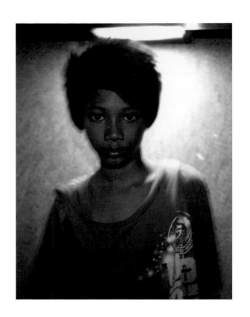

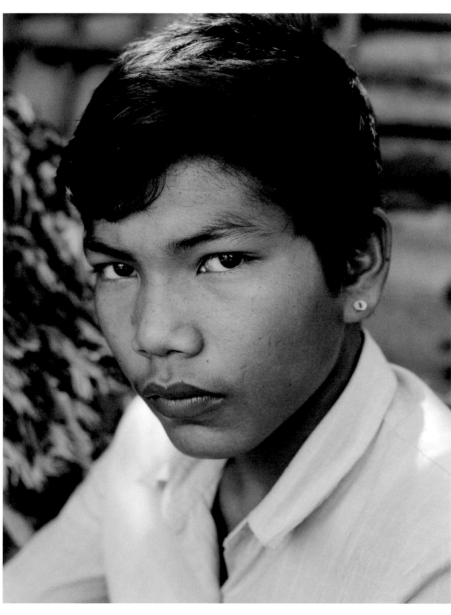

Chardchakaj Waikawee

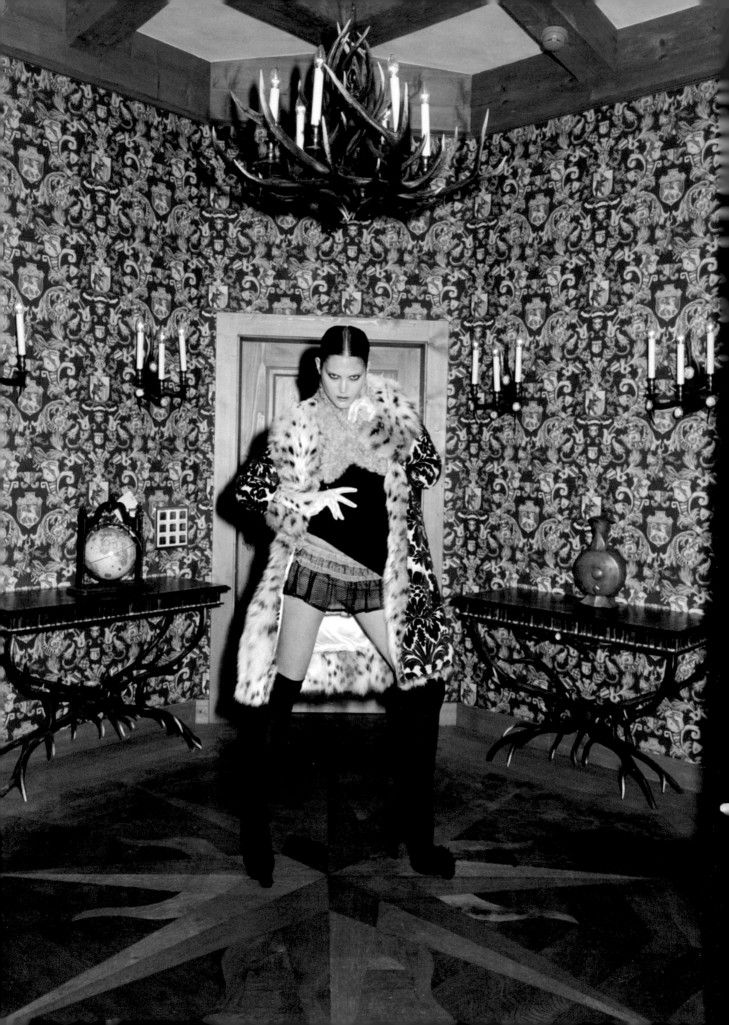

Tung Walsh makes vivid, energetic and often theatrical colour photographs.

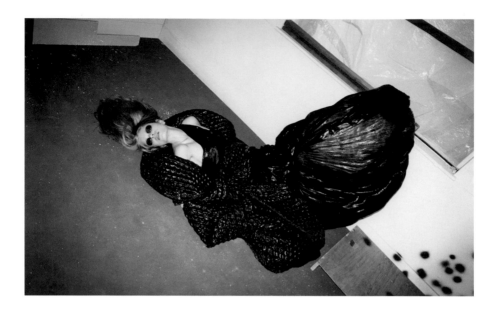

British photographer Tung Walsh (b. 1976) started out as a darkroom technician at the London College of Printing (now London College of Communication) in the early 2000s. While there, he observed that photography students, who at the time were around his own age, were going on to take up positions as assistants to well-known fashion photographers. In 2001, after winning a competition held at London's Photographers' Gallery, and upon discovering a library book on Juergen Teller, he wrote to the German photographer to ask for work. Not long after, he was contacted by the late Katy Baggott, Teller's long-time agent and producer, and a highly regarded and influential figure in the industry, and offered the job. For the next five years, Walsh worked closely with Teller and Baggott as the photographer's only assistant. It was a formative experience that ultimately launched his career in fashion photography.

Walsh makes vivid, energetic colour photographs, working predominantly on film with a hand-held camera.

Environmental portraiture is an important strand of his editorial output, and he has published portraits of the architects Rem Koolhaas and Zaha Hadid, as well as the artists Gilbert and George, and Jeff Koons. His photographs consciously reference the aesthetic of spontaneous 'point-and-shoot' image-making, as well as recent 'realist' work by photographers such as Walter Pfeiffer, Terry Richardson and, of course, Teller. In its confrontation with or celebration of a strong, sometimes sexual femininity and irreverent or humorous approach to the medium, we could also compare Walsh's work to that of Helmut Newton. While Walsh's images of models hanging out on the street, at the seaside or in American-style diners and Chinese restaurants are very much of the moment, they also evoke the nostalgic glamour found in late 1970s and early '80s work by Newton and other photographers such as Jeanloup Sieff and Guy Bourdin.

Walsh received his first commission from *Dazed & Confused*'s photography editor Emma Reeves and shortly after started working with *i-D*'s former art director Dean Langley.

He has also collaborated extensively with the stylist Tamara Rothstein. His images are frequently shot on location and these different settings are an integral part of the compositions. Often architectural quirks or elaborate ornamentation – intricate wood panelling, lavishly patterned carpets and wallpapers, grandiose chandeliers or lush gardens – create a heightened sense of theatricality and even absurdity when used as a backdrop to a sequence of images. Elsewhere, lo-fi settings – motel rooms or sparsely carpeted sets – contrast with the bold prints and extravagant trimmings of the high-fashion garments on display.

Walsh has contributed to a range of publications: *Self Service, Pop, Arena Homme+, Industrie, 032c, W, V, Russh, T: The New York Times Style Magazine, Wall Street Journal, Smithsonian, Hercules, Tar, The Sunday Times Magazine, The Sunday Times Style, Times Luxx* and *Süddeutsche Zeitung*. His commercial clients include Moncler, Costume National, Dolce & Gabbana, Nike, Fred Perry, Martine Rose, Topshop, Asos and Bon Marché.

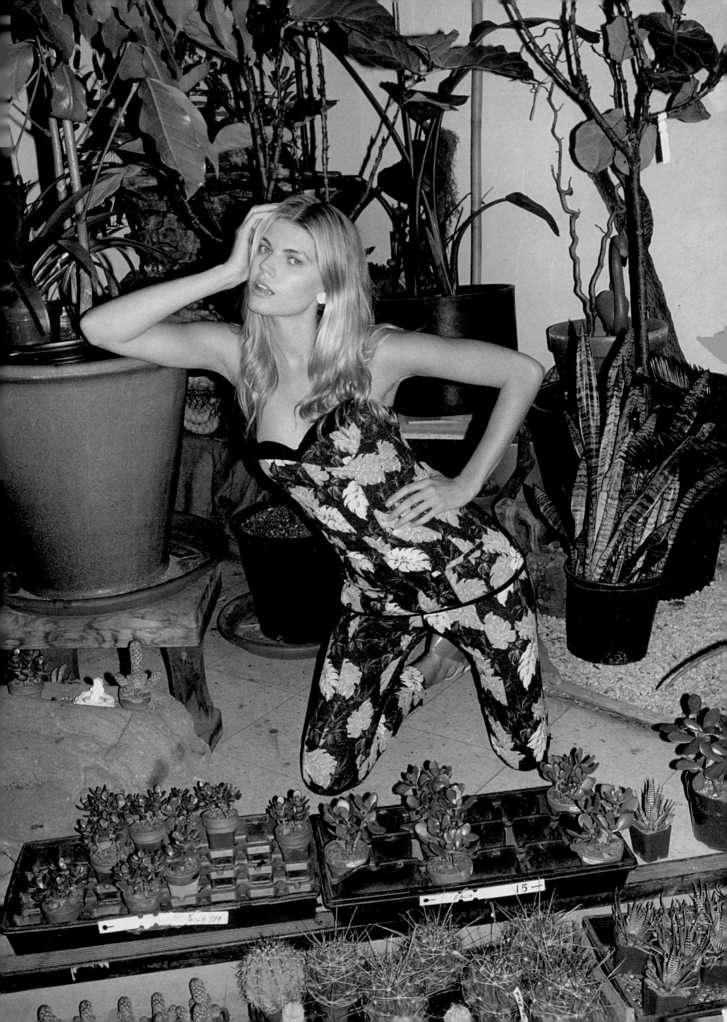

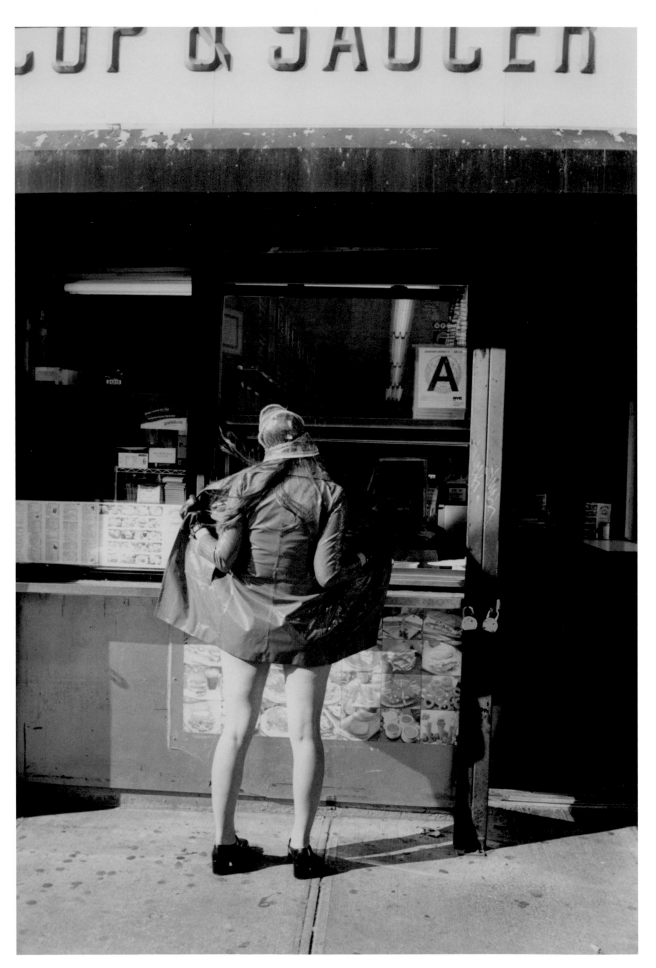

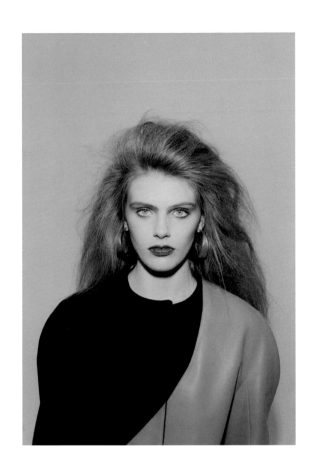

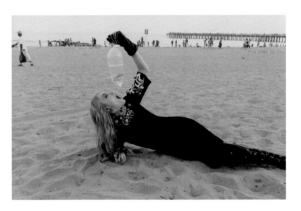

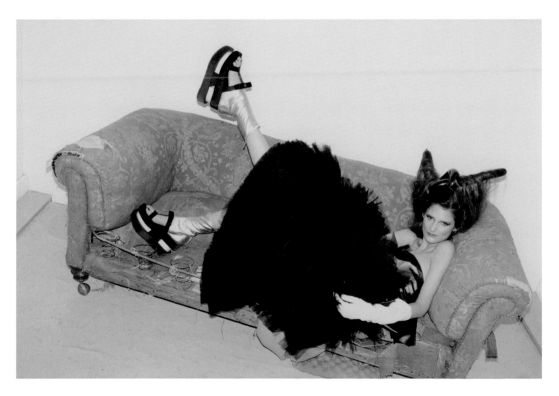

Tung Walsh

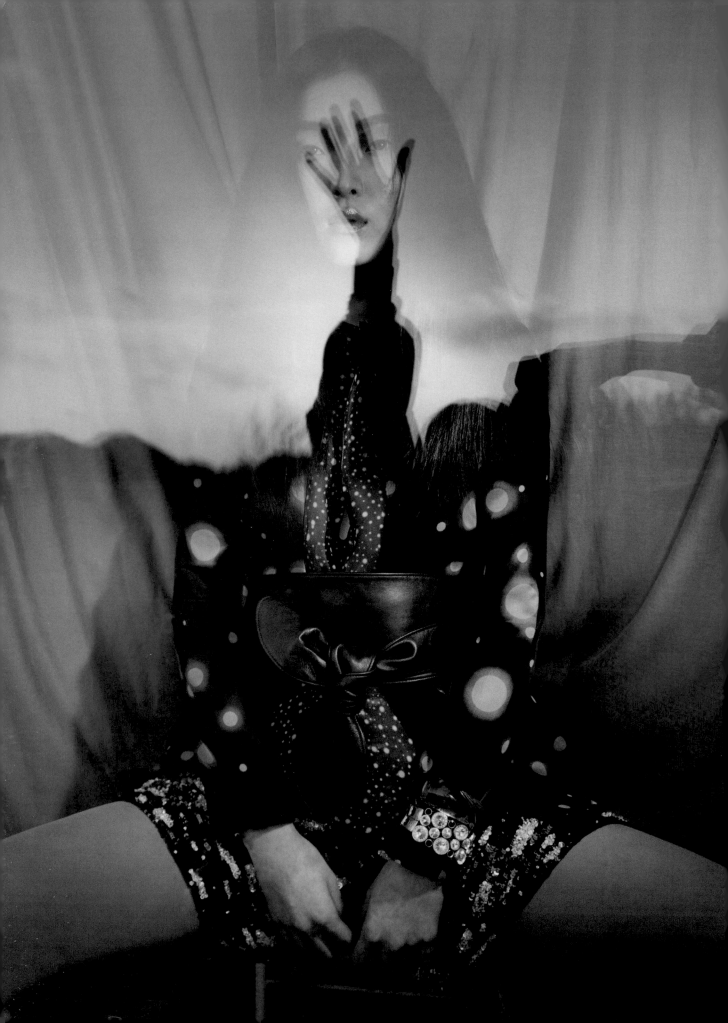

Harley Weir's work displays a flexibility of technique, casting and conceptualization.

Harley Weir

———

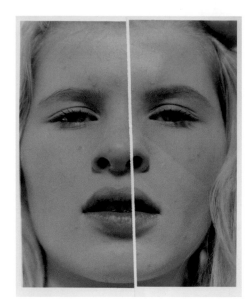

Harley Weir (b. 1988) is a London-based photographer. She graduated from Central Saint Martins College of Art and Design with a degree in fine art in 2010. Weir taught herself photography by regularly taking pictures of her family and friends in and around West London and then developing and manipulating the negatives at home. Much has been made of the new opportunities offered by digital platforms and the capacity of the internet to provide emerging photographers with an entry into fashion editorial. Weir posted her images on Flickr, where they were noticed and subsequently published by *Vice*. Since then, her work has appeared in numerous magazines, including *AnOther*, *Under/Current*, *Dazed & Confused*, *b Store*, *Citizen K* and *Grit*, as well as on websites such as *i-D* online.

Weir often works on location with natural light. Her images are diaristic and her approach to her subjects and their environment is portrait-based. Within this, the fashion garments help to build up a strong sense of character: even when styled, they seem to belong to Weir's sitters as parts of a life well lived. Certainly in her early work, this could be seen as an extension of her own life and experiences. Texture – flowers, fabrics, or the patterns found in shadows and effects of light – has remained another important preoccupation. Weir often creates surface patterns by marking or drawing on her negatives and prints. Many of her pictures feature small lines repeated at intervals: these are sometimes used as a compositional device – layered, say, over a studio portrait set against a plain background – while in other cases the marks suggest a certain aura or energy surrounding the image subject.

Like many of the photographers in this book, Weir is not restricted by the traditional definition of fashion imagery, nor does she follow any predetermined 'guidelines' on how to make fashion pictures. Instead, her work displays a flexibility of technique, casting and conceptualization. Weir photographs male and female subjects with equal confidence and subtlety, and embraces the range of possibilities offered by both digital and analogue formats: double exposures; drawing and hand tinting; printing and rephotographing digital prints; and digital post-production. She abandons the extreme, almost alien or androgynous perfection and seamless retouching that was perpetuated by the brand advertising and fashion editorials published in the 'super glossies' during the early 2000s. Once again, this creative freedom is a result of the resurgence of independent magazines and small-scale self-publishing, with art directors and editors now willing to commission photographers such as Weir who extend current conventions or experiment with new directions.

———

254 'Untitled', *AnOther*, 2012 — 256 'Beth', 2013 — 257 'Harry', *Citizen K*, 2011
258 'Isaac', *Husk*, 2011 — 259 above 'Israel / Palestine', *GUP*, 2013 — 259 below 'Grace', *Baron*, 2013

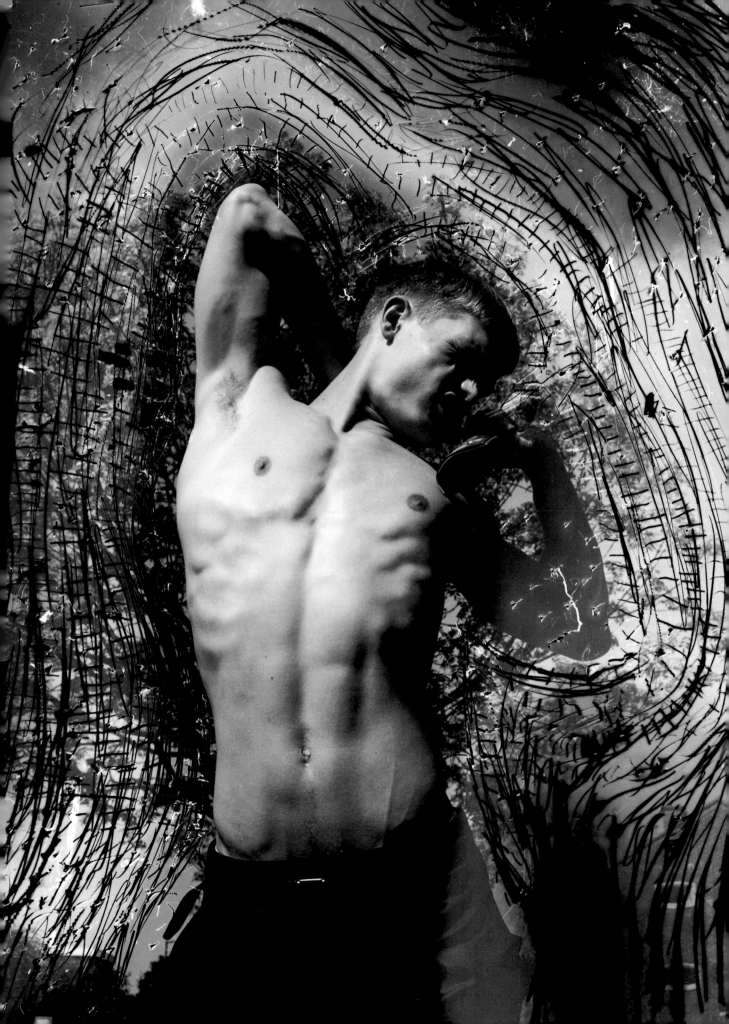

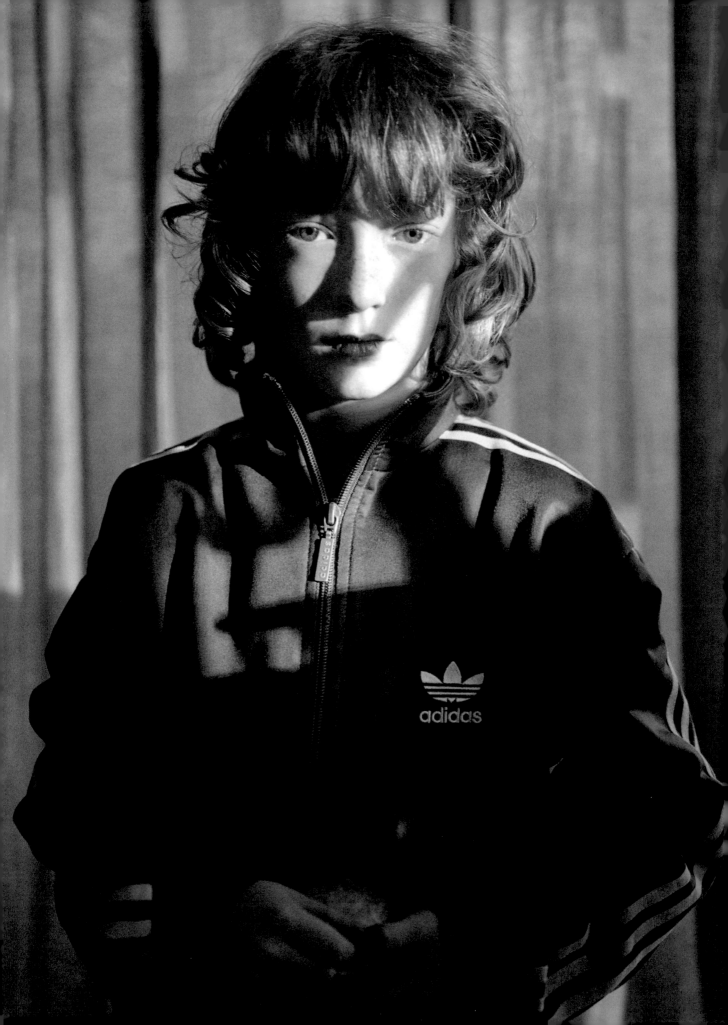

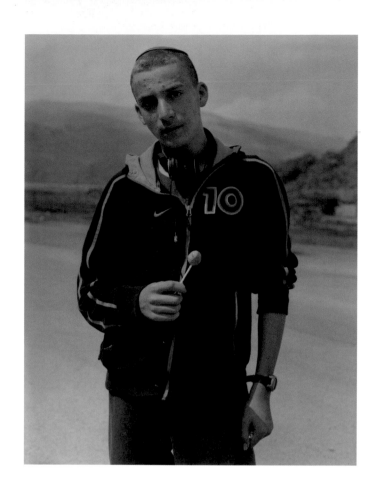

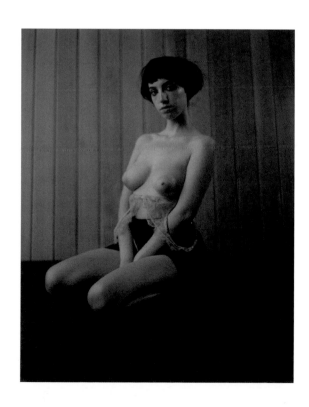

Harley Weir

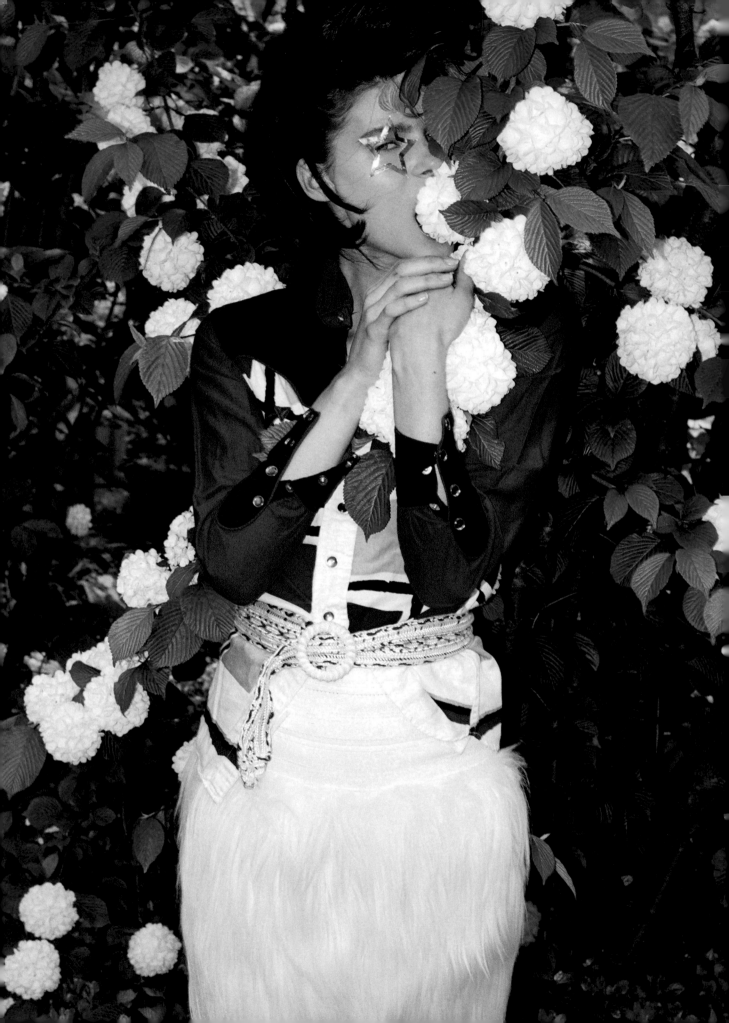

Ruvan Wijesooriya is an inquisitive photographer who is attracted to absurd situations.

Ruvan Wijesooriya

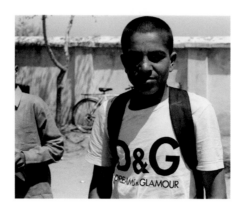

Ruvan Wijesooriya (b. 1977) was born in Duluth, Minnesota, the son of Sri Lankan immigrants. He studied sociology, anthropology, political economy and gender studies at Lewis & Clark College in Portland, Oregon. Shortly after graduating in 1999, he moved to New York, where he has since been based.

Wijesooriya has no formal photographic training but came to the medium via his interest in music and work as a music journalist and stylist in the early 2000s. During this period he would sometimes take photographs of the musicians he was writing about, and eventually the shooting took over. These days his practice spans music, fashion, art, travel and documentary. Although this may seem inconsistent, Wijesooriya's diligence while shooting and editing ensures that none of his images is superfluous.

Approximately 85 per cent of Wijesooriya's photographs are made on film, although he uses many different cameras to achieve his very distinctive, usually high-contrast look. He often carries a small automatic analogue Pentax on his person in case something occurs that needs to be recorded. An inquisitive photographer with a quirky sense of humour, he is attracted to absurd situations – an old lady hunched under an umbrella with a Chanel carrier bag stuffed with plastic, for instance – and often constructs strange scenarios himself with the help of props or by extracting unexpected expressions from his subjects. When it comes to his fashion photography, he believes that everyone knows that models are physically beautiful, so instead tries to capture the beauty of their personalities. This explains why many of his images have a playful, cheeky or ironic quality, and even feature smiling models. Wijesooriya often arranges his pictures in groups of seemingly unrelated images. By collaging together different photographs or placing them next to each other, or by juxtaposing still-life, fashion, portrait, music or documentary images, he allows new relations to emerge between the genres.

Wijesooriya's work has been published in numerous magazines: *The New Yorker*, British and Italian *Vogue*, US *Nylon*, *Flair*, *L'Officiel*, *A4*, *Dazed & Confused* and *Rolling Stone*, to name a few. He has worked for the fashion designers Jill Stuart and Paul Smith, as well as the music labels EMI and DFA Records, photographing acts such as LCD Soundsystem, Iggy Pop, The Rapture and Blood Orange, among others. The hit American television series *Gossip Girl* based a character on Wijesooriya and used ten of his fine-art prints to decorate the permanent set. He has also shown work at exhibitions and music festivals in the USA, Sweden, the UK, Spain and France. His publications include *All Night New York*, a collection of black-and-white photographs documenting the New York night life released in 2008.

Wijesooriya moved around a lot as a child and periods of his adult life have been spent in the UK and Sweden. He often travels even further afield for his photography: in 2011 he went to Afghanistan where he took the picture 'Dreams and Glamour' of a boy in a faux Dolce & Gabbana T-shirt. His oeuvre is testament to a life of movement – an accumulation of photographs of the people he meets, the places he goes and the experiences he has along the way. The overriding sentiment here is generous rather than opportunistic, however. For example, visitors to 'Dearest Of Dearest', his 2011 exhibition of personal work at Ion Studio in New York, were able to take home the 6×4 inch prints on display without paying a cent, providing they left notes on the wall in the place of the photographs. This was a warm gesture in the spirit of exchange on Wijesooriya's part: it acknowledged the role played both by his close friends and the world at large in the realization of his projects. The show was a novel way of stimulating an engagement with photography that is not based on the need to purchase a fetishized object, nor on the need to surf the internet.

---

260 'Pollen', *A4*, 2008 — **262** 'Dreams and Glamour', 2011 — **263** 'Malin out of the Window', *Odd At Large*, 2007 — **264** 'Purple Dress (Sculptural)', *A4*, 2008
265 above 'Untitled (Kim in Bathtub with Snorkel Mask)', 2008 — **265 below** 'Untitled (Future Fashion Wasteland)', *Twelv*, 2012
266 'Anouck with red background', *L'Officiel* (Belgium), 2009 — **267** 'Chanel on 26th Street', 2006

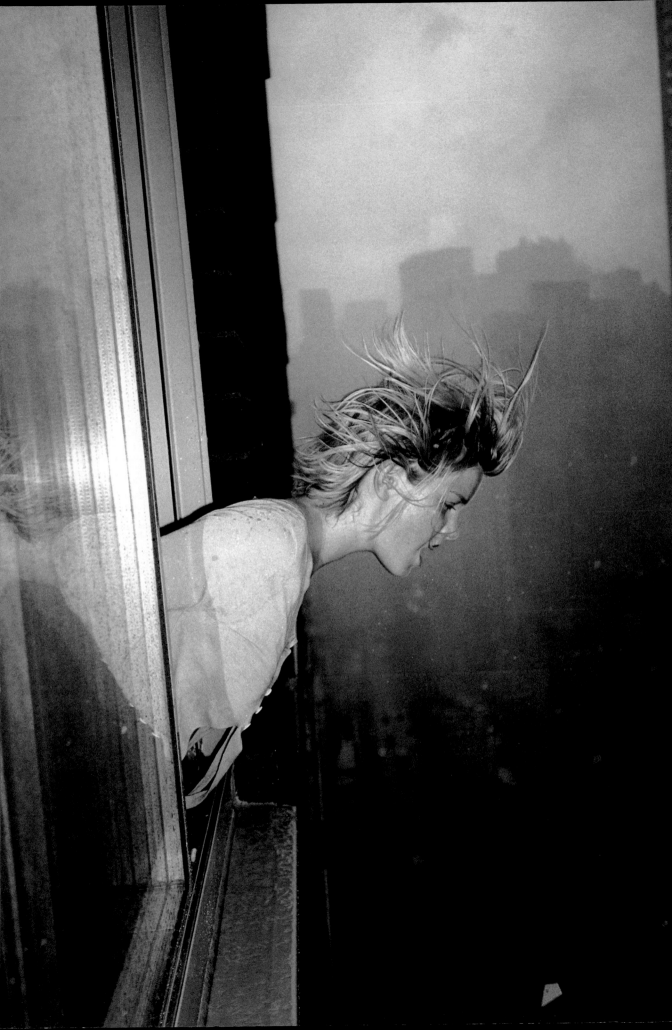

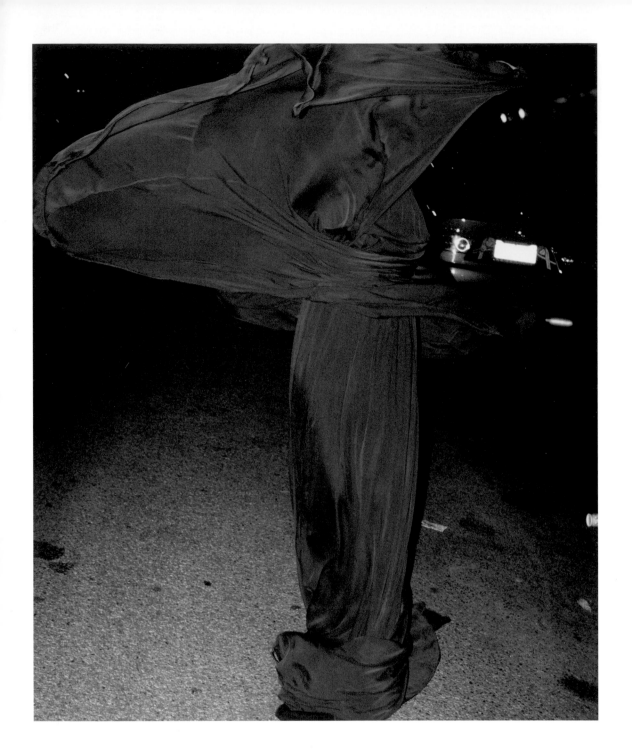

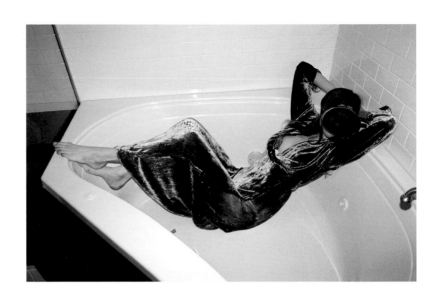

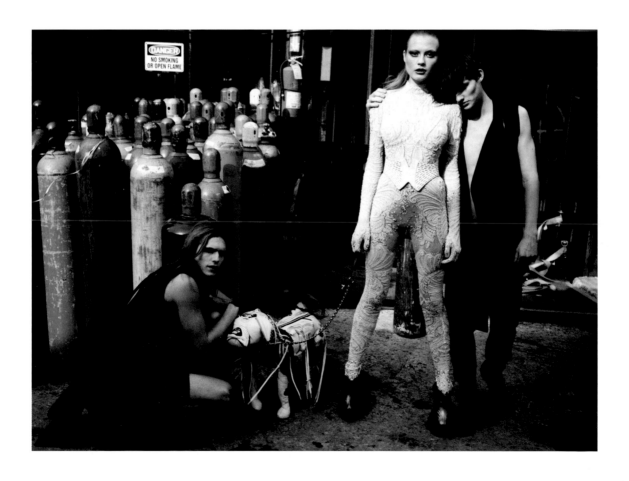

Ruvan Wijesooriya

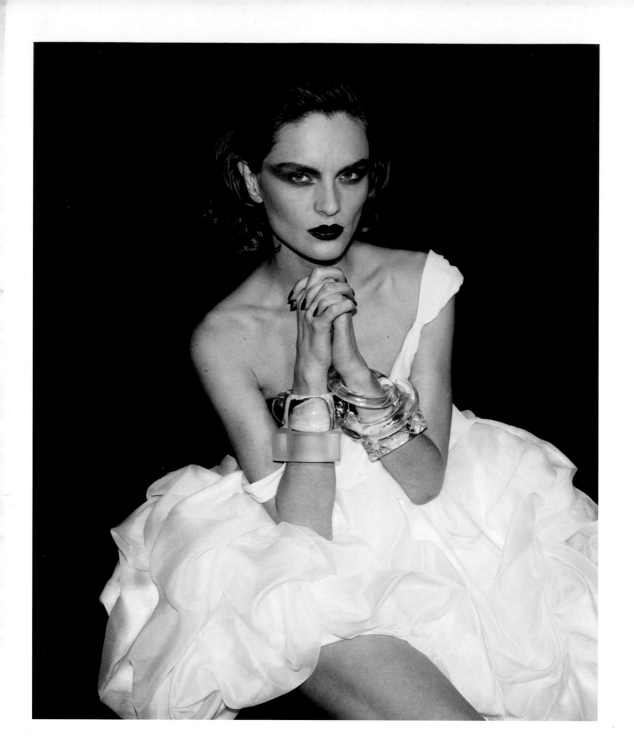

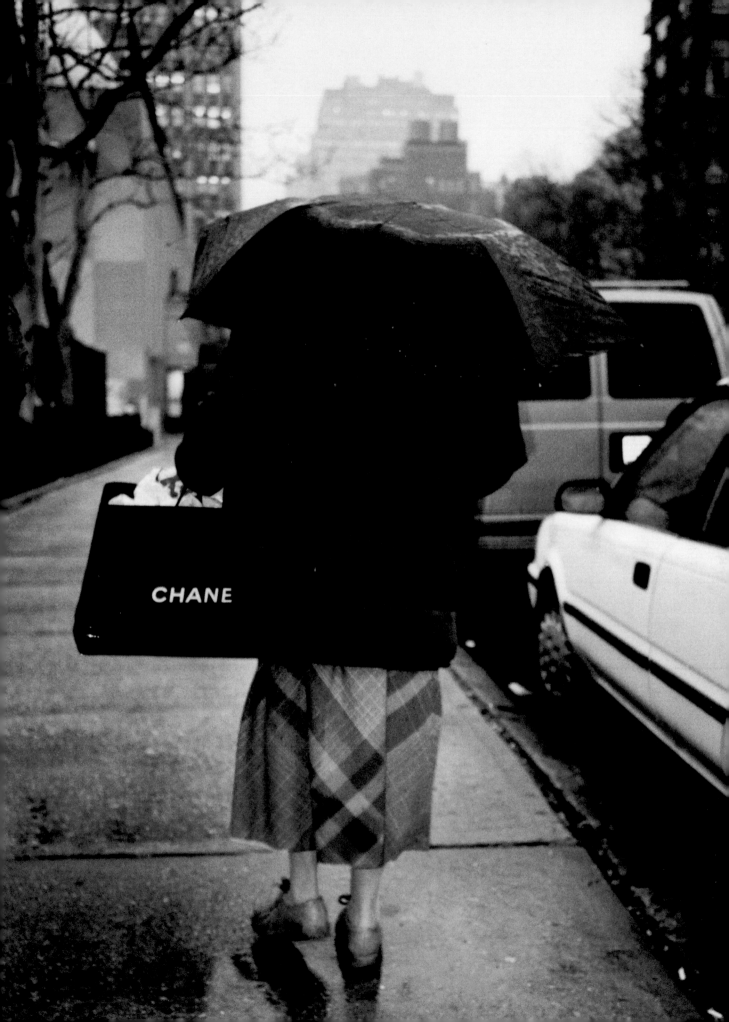

Marion de Beaupré et al. (eds)
Archeology of Elegance, 1980–2000:
20 Years of Fashion Photography
London: Thames & Hudson, 2002

Susan Bright
Face of Fashion
London: National Portrait Gallery,
2007

Stella Bruzzi and Pamela Church
Gibson (eds)
Fashion Cultures: Theories,
Explorations and Analysis
London: Routledge, 2001

Charlotte Cotton
Imperfect Beauty: The Making of
Contemporary Fashion Photographs
London: V&A Publications, 2000

Robin Derrick and Robin Muir (eds)
Unseen Vogue: The Secret History
of Fashion Photography
London: Little, Brown, 2002

Jason Evans (ed.)
W'Happen
London: Shoreditch Biennale, 1998

Jefferson Hack
Another Fashion Book
Göttingen: Steidl, 2009

Jefferson Hack and Jo-Ann Furniss (eds)
Dazed & Confused: Making It Up As
We Go Along: A Visual History Of
The Magazine That Broke All The Rules
New York: Rizzoli, 2011

Susan Gaensheimer and Sophie von
Olfers (eds)
Not in Fashion: Photography and
Fashion in the 90s
Bielefeld: Kerber, 2011

Nancy Hall-Duncan
The History of Fashion Photography
New York: Alpine Book Co., 1979

Martin Harrison
Appearances: Fashion Photography
Since 1945
London: Jonathan Cape, 1991

Nathalie Herschdorfer
Coming into Fashion: A Century
of Photography at Condé Nast
London: Thames & Hudson, 2012

Terry Jones
30 Years of i-D
London: Taschen, 2010

Susan Kismaric and Eva Repini
Fashioning Fiction in Photography
Since 1990
New York: Museum of Modern Art,
2004

Alexander Liberman
The Art and Technique of
Color Photography
New York: Simon & Schuster, 1951

Eugénie Shinkle (ed.)
Fashion as Photograph:
Viewing and Reviewing Images
of Fashion
London: I.B. Tauris, 2008

Mark C. Taylor
Hiding
University of Chicago Press, 1997

Val Williams
Look at Me: Fashion Photography
in Britain, 1960 to the Present
London: British Council, 1998

Acknowledgments

———

I would first like to thank the photographers featured in this book.
All were patient and supportive over a long period of research and writing, and all
have shown great generosity in a myriad of ways, making this project a reality and a joy.

Thanks must go to my commissioning editor at Thames & Hudson, Andrew Sanigar;
to Tatiana Goodchild; Jane Cutter; and especially to my editor, Theresa Morgan,
who worked with great care and dedication on refining the texts.
Thanks also to the team at Barnbrook for designing the book.

I would like to thank Eleanor Weber, my co-contributor, whose commitment,
writing and incredible sensitivity have made this book infinitely better than
anything I could have produced alone.

Special thanks to Julie Brown, one of the most influential and brilliant figures in
contemporary fashion photography, whose knowledge and perspective has contributed greatly
to my research for this book and enabled so much of my work.

I would also like to specially thank eX de Medici for helping me to proceed
in the best way possible and for keeping me writing.

For professional, creative and intellectual contributions, thank you to:
Bruno Ceschel, Self Publish, Be Happy; Professor Frances Corner, Head of College, London College of Fashion
and Ligaya Salazar, Director, Fashion Space Gallery; Neil Hobbs and Karina Harris;
Claudia Küssell, Curator at Foam Fotografiemuseum Amsterdam;
Marco Santucci, Santucci & Co.; Victoria Sullivan and Joe Streeter, Streeters;
Shawn Waldron, Senior Director, Archives and Records, Condé Nast and Brett Croft, British *Vogue*;
Jules Wright, The Wapping Project Bankside; and my colleagues at the Centre for Art History
and Art Theory at the Australian National University.

Writing over two continents and two years, I would have given it all up without
Mark and Rachael Bray, Susan Bright, Jane Cassidy, Rae Chittock, Charlotte Cotton,
Mark Dyson, Helen Ennis, Jordan Evans-Tse, Nathan Firth, Sally Gray, Heidi Grivas,
David Head, Ben Hehir, Erin Hinton, Anthony Luvera, Rae Chittock, Penny Martin,
Gregorio Pagliaro, Katrina Power, Giles Price, Tom Pye, Rebecca Roberts, Andrew Sayers,
Louise Shannon, Eleanor Struth and Jesse Whyte.

Final thanks must go to my incredibly supportive siblings, and to Irfan Master.

This book is for Dr Margaret-O'Flynn Keaney AM and Dr James Keaney AM.
Quod scripsi, scripsi.

———

Magda Keaney

Page numbers in italic refer to illustrations

Index